Hair Structure and Chemistry Simplified

Hair Structure and Chemistry Simplified

Fourth Edition

John Halal

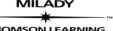

MILADY
™
THOMSON LEARNING

Australia Canada Mexico Singapore Spain United Kingdom United States

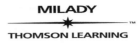

MILADY
★
™
THOMSON LEARNING

Hair Structure and Chemistry Simplified, Fourth Edition
by John Halal

MILADY STAFF:
President:
Susan L. Simpfenderfer

Publisher:
Marlene McHugh Pratt

Acquisitions Editor:
Pamela B. Lappies

Developmental Editor:
Judy Roberts

Executive Production Manager:
Wendy A. Troeger

Production Editor:
Eileen M. Clawson

Text Design and Composition:
Carlisle Publishers Services

Executive Marketing Manager:
Donna J. Lewis

Channel Manager:
Wendy Mapstone

Cover Design:
Dutton and Sherman Design

For more information contact Milady, 3 Columbia Circle, PO Box 15015, Albany, NY 12212-5015
Or find us on the World Wide Web at http://www.milady.com
For permission to use material from this text or product, contact us by
Tel (800) 730-2214   Fax (800) 730-2215   www.thomsonrights.com

Library of Congress Cataloging-in-Publication Data
Halal, John.
   Hair structure and chemistry simplified / John Halal.—4th ed., rev.
      p. cm.
   Rev. ed. of: Milady's hair structure and chemistry simplified / Douglas D. Schoon. 1993.
   ISBN 1-56253-629-X
   1. Hairdressing. 2. Hair—Care and hygiene. I. Schoon, Douglas D. Milady's hair
structure and chemistry simplified. II. Title.
   TT972 .H33 2001
   646.7′24—dc21

                                                                      2001028139

This book is dedicated to my wife, Marty,
and my daughters, Heather and Allison.

Table of Contents

Preface

Although chemistry is an essential part of everything that a professional hairstylist does, few have any real knowledge about the chemicals in the products they use or the countless chemical reactions that take place in a salon each day. In addition to the dangers to the hairstylist and the client, this lack of knowledge also limits the hairstylist's ability and perpetuates a negative image of hairstyling as a profession.

Most hairstylists are intimidated by chemistry because it's usually presented with formulas, chemical symbols, and long unpronounceable words that seem to be written in some exotic, foreign language. Old wives' tales and exaggerated marketing claims further confuse students by adding a wealth of misinformation, which may be easy to understand but is all too often incorrect. *Hair Structure and Chemistry Simplified, Fourth Edition* separates fact from fiction and clears up the confusion. The direct approach of this text overcomes the apprehension usually associated with learning chemistry. Hairstylists will find the information easy to understand and even easier to use. The easy to apply concepts presented in this text will empower hairstylists with understanding that will improve both the quality and the safety of their salon services.

Recent advances in cosmetic chemistry have transformed yesterday's hairdressers and barbers into today's hi-tech hairstylists. The traditional cold wave has a variety of new replacements. Hairstylists must now choose between acid, exothermic, no ammonia, no thio, and self-timing permanents. Old-fashioned hair dyes have been replaced with semi-permanent, demi-permanent and para-permanent hair colorants. Herbal powdered hair lighteners have replaced bleach and enzyme developers substitute for peroxide. Chemical services in today's modern salons have been turbocharged with high volumes of peroxide, chemical catalysts and color processing machines.

But all of these new products may not live up to their promises. Some can be dangerous, and some cost more—much more. Are they really worth the additional expense? Are they safe? How is a hairstylist to know which product to use and how to use that product safely? *Hair Structure and Chemistry Simplified, Fourth Edition*, helps students, as well as experienced hairstylists, select the right product from the flood of new products that were not available a few short years ago.

Learning the language of cosmetic chemistry, presented in this text, empowers hairstylists with an understanding of what's actually in those bottles and why it's there. With a little practice, hairstylists will learn to read and translate the ingredients listed, in small print, on the back of the bottle. Those who don't understand the language are relegated to reading only the exaggerated marketing claims prominently listed, in big print, on the front of the bottle.

Most hairstylists have little difficulty learning the intimate details of the mechanical tools of their trade: scissors, brushes, hot irons, and hairdryers. This revision applies that same level of understanding to their chemical tools: haircolorants, permanent wave solutions, chemical hair relaxers, chemical depilatories, shampoos, conditioners, styling aids, and sunscreens. Although these tools are every bit as important, they are usually less understood.

Hair Structure and Chemistry Simplified, Fourth Edition, is the most current, comprehensive and straightforward textbook of its kind. This text thoroughly explains the theory and application of many essential concepts that are simply not covered in other texts. New material has been added which includes the new products and services that are currently being performed in today's modern salons.

This revision has also eliminated some outdated material without sacrificing the integrity of the original text. Many photographs, drawings, and line art have been replaced with clearer images and better illustrations. New artwork has also been added that improves the visual representation of essential ideas.

The Glossary and Index has been expanded and the Appendix now includes information on product labeling along with samples of Material Safety Data Sheets and lists of product ingredients. A complete list of Key Terms has been added to the beginning of each chapter.

New material, not found in other texts, boldly presents the concept, importance, and relevance of pH in cosmetics. The section on emulsions and surfactants explains the dynamics of surface tension and distinguishes between the hydrophobic and hydrophilic properties essential for all emulsions. Advanced information on multiple phase and microemulsions (liposomes and nanospheres) is also included. The benefits and dangers of exposure to ultraviolet light are discussed, along with an explanation of sunscreens, Sun Protection Factor, and the new Federal Drug Administration monograph, which details their use. This book also draws attention to the dangers of mixing different chemicals, even those that may seem completely safe.

Hair Structure and Chemistry Simplified, Fourth Edition, will improve student comprehension and retention and provide graduates with a valuable resource to aid them throughout their career. Even the most experienced hairstylists will gain confidence and control as they learn to make intelligent, informed decisions about the chemical services they perform everyday in the salon. This text helps hairstylists avoid problems before they start and shows them how to correct small problems before they become big problems.

A complete supplement package, which has been updated to correspond with the revisions of the text, complements and reinforces all the key ideas.

Exam Review, ISBN: 1-56253-631-1. The Exam Review reinforces the text and permits instructors to monitor student learning easily. These multiple-choice questions quickly allow teachers to determine exactly which concepts have been learned and which still need attention. Answers are provided with the text, which allow for self-review and student practice.

Workbook, ISBN: 1-56253-630-3. The workbook questions are designed to provide a student activity that stimulates student thinking and expands the ideas presented in the text. Students learn to organize ideas and differentiate key points. Many of the questions in the workbook require answers in essay form.

Course Management Guide, ISBN: 1-56253-632-X. This consists of four sections that enable instructors to explore the text material with added confidence and in greater detail.

1. Answers to Workbook. Clear, concise answers clarify the concepts presented in the Workbook and facilitate grading by the instructor. These answers are not found in the workbook.

2. Answers to Textbook Review and Discussion Questions. Provides complete answers to the Review and Discussion Questions at the end of each chapter in the textbook. These answers are not found in the textbook.

3. Lectures and Lesson Plans. This section complements and expands the textbook. Instructors will find the in-depth information invaluable in the preparation of lectures and the presentation of key ideas that are presented in the textbook.

4. Classroom Experiments. These safe, simple experiments permit teachers to create unforgettable moments of learning that bring chemistry to life for students and instructors. When performed by the teacher as a presentation, these experiments grab and hold student attention. Many of the experiments are so simple, safe, and easy to do that supervised students can work in small groups, monitoring and recording their own progress.

ABOUT THE AUTHOR

John Halal began his career as a hairstylist over 30 years ago. In addition to John & Friends, Inc., his two successful salons in suburban Indianapolis, he also owns and operates International Concepts Beauty Supply and Honors Beauty College, Inc.

Halal is an active member of the National Cosmetology Association (NCA), the Salon Association (TSA), the Indiana Cosmetology Educators Association (ICEA), the American Association of Cosmetology Schools (AACS), the Beauty & Barber Supply Institute (BBSI), and the Society of Cosmetic Chemists (SCC).

John & Friends, Inc., was featured as the *Salon of the Month* by *American Salon Magazine* and has been selected, for the past three consecutive years, as one of *America's Top 200 Fastest Growing Salons* by *Salon Today Magazine*. John and

Friends, Inc., also received the Reader's Choice Award for *Best Salon* from Indianapolis Monthly Magazine. Halal's essay, *What a Difference a Decade Makes*, was chosen as one of the *Outstanding Call for Presentation Papers* by the BBSI. His classroom presentation received the award for *Outstanding Educational Program* from the Indiana State Cosmetologist Association.

Halal obtained his associate's degree, with highest distinction, from Indiana University and is currently completing his bachelor's. He has authored articles on a wide variety of topics and has been published in several professional trade magazines. He often travels, as a guest speaker, to address professional and consumer groups.

ACKNOWLEDGMENTS

I would like to thank the following individuals and companies who provided information and helped me with the research for this book. I wish to express my gratitude for their help.

Dr. Martin J. O'Donnell, Department of Chemistry, Indiana University, IN

Keith C. Brown, Ph.D., Director of Research Worldwide Beauty Care, Bristol Myers Squibb

TRI, Institute of Trichology.

REVIEWERS

I would also like to thank the following cosmetology professionals for their assistance and expertise in the preparation of this revision and reviewing the final manuscript.

Sharon S. Aresco, Vinal Technical High School, Middletown, CT

Sharon K. Barnard, KACC School of Cosmetology, Milford, IL

Kenneth W. Dennis, Alternative Hair Clinic, Columbia, SC

Cheryl Goostree, Univ School of Hair Technology, Bowling Green, KY

Patricia Martin, International School of Beauty, Inc., New Port Richey, FL

Robert Morey, Flint Institute of Barbering Inc., Flint, MI

Robin Ratliff, Gainesville School of Hairstyling, Gainesville, FL

Kerry Stroman, College of Hair Design, Lincoln, NE

Madeline Udod, Eastern Suffolk BOCES, Bellport, NY

Betty Walker, Carolina Academy, Gastonia, NC

Beth Wallace, Northwest-Shoals Community College, Phil Campbell, AL

Chapter 1

Science and Cosmetology

Learning Objectives

After completing this chapter, you should be able to:

- Understand what science is and is not.

- Use the three basic steps of the scientific method to improve learning.

- Explain the "cause-and-effect" relationship and its importance.

- Understand the difference between safe and dangerous experimentation.

- Distinguish between scientific breakthroughs and marketing sales tools.

- Find other sources of information and continuing education.

CHEMISTRY IN THE SALON

"Why should I study chemistry? I want to learn hairstyling, not chemistry." If you're like most hairstylists, you love learning about all the artistic aspects of hairstyling and can't wait for your next haircutting class. And although haircutting may seem much more important than chemistry, if you intend to shampoo, condition, color, perm, or relax hair successfully, chemistry is every bit as important.

What would happen if you didn't understand the inherent difference between a razor haircut and a scissor haircut? How would you decide which tool to use? Without an understanding of the geometry of a haircut how would you know the correct angles to hold and cut the hair? Imagine what would happen if you had to perform a haircut in the dark and couldn't see the hair or the scissors?

These may seem like extreme examples, but they aren't really. Hairstylists who perform chemical services without understanding the basic chemistry involved do not understand the chemical tools they are using. They are unable to "see" clearly what they are doing. It's not that different from cutting hair in the dark. In both cases, they are flying blind and are forced to rely on guesswork. Not being able to clearly see lowers the quality of salon services and causes inconsistent and erratic results. Nothing is worse than being lost in the dark and unable to see the way out.

Although the same level of excitement that's associated with hairstyling isn't usually attached to chemistry, there's no reason it can't be. With a basic understanding of salon chemistry, you will be able to select the right haircolor or permanent wave for even the most difficult client. You will be able to predict the results ahead of time accurately, the first time and every time. You will be able to identify and avoid most problems long before they become big problems. When problems do arise, you will be able to correct them quickly and easily with the confidence that comes from knowing. With a basic understanding of salon chemistry, you can eliminate guesswork, dissatisfied clients, and those recurring problems that just never seem to get resolved.

WHAT IS SCIENCE?

The word **science** is derived from the Latin *scientia*, meaning "knowledge." Science is the pursuit of knowledge about the universe around us. Scientific knowledge involves the ability to explain established facts, in terms of a physical cause for an observed effect. Chemistry, biology, physics, and geometry are examples of different kinds of science. In this book, we will study the science of chemistry.

WHAT IS CHEMISTRY?

Chemistry is the study of matter and its changes. Matter is the material and structure of the universe. Everything that we see, touch, taste, and smell is made of matter. Chemistry is often referred to as the "central science" because chemistry is essential to all other sciences.

WHAT IS TECHNOLOGY?

Technology is the use of scientific knowledge to manipulate nature. Technology provides hairstylists with all the tools used in a modern salon. You are probably familiar with physical styling tools, which create physical changes and include scissors, brushes, combs, hot irons, and hairdryers. Hairstylists also use chemical tools, which create chemical changes and include permanent wave solutions, haircolorants, hair relaxers, and chemical depilatories. Hairstyling would not be possible without science, chemistry, and technology.

THE SCIENTIFIC METHOD

The **scientific method** is a term used to describe the methodology of science. It is how science is done. This logical, objective approach to solving problems is based on three major steps:

1. **Observation**—Gathering facts by experimentation
2. **Reasoning**—Speculation or idea that explains the observation
3. **Testing**—Further experimentation to test and retest the idea

Observation

All learning is done through observation. You use observation every day in the salon when you evaluate the results of the services you perform. When a permanent wave turns out curlier than expected or a haircolor ends up darker than you thought it would be, you observed the results of your own experiments. If something goes wrong, the scientific method will help you to figure out what went wrong and how to correct the problem.

Accurate, detailed, systematic recordkeeping is essential to objective observation and the application of the scientific method. The purpose of observation is the collection of facts and the arrangement of those facts into a pattern that reveals the reason for the observed results. The importance of accurate records cannot be overemphasized. Hairstylists that fall victim to the dangers of bad record-keeping are forever doomed to repeat past mistakes.

Client records should include a complete evaluation of the length, texture, color, and condition of the hair, prior to the service and the results that are expected. Extra caution should be used to determine any previous problems or adverse reactions the client may have had in the past. This information must be reevaluated prior to each service since there may have been a change in the client's history or in the formulation of the product since it was last used. Also include in your records the method of application, the formula, processing time, and the results achieved.

OBSERVATION EXPERIMENT

As you read this page, most of the information collected by your eyes and ears is unconsciously filtered out and ignored. Try the following experiment and see how much you're missing.

Don't move your head or eyes from this page. Now concentrate on seeing the edges of the book while you continue to read. Now expand your vision awareness outward and see just what else your brain has been hiding as you read. Can you see your wrist, your arms, the floor, or walls? Now listen carefully—are there any sounds in the background that you didn't notice before? Do they sound a little different when you concentrate on them?

Your brain protects you from a constant battering of sights and sounds. It would be hard to live in today's world of noise and confusion if we had to see and hear *everything*. However, we must not allow our brains to get lazy; the brain may block out too much important information. Being more observant is simply paying closer attention. It is a way of telling the brain to notice more of what our eyes and ears are telling us.

Reasoning

The fastest, most powerful computers in the world cannot match a human's ability to reason. When you use any information to reach a conclusion or make a decision, you are using the **power of reasoning.** Reasoning turns observations into useful ideas. Reasoning increases your product knowledge and improves your techniques. Nothing will help you more in developing a successful cosmetology career than using your vast power of reason. If you keep accurate records and the results you observe weren't what you expected, you can use your power of reasoning to figure out why. Once you've determined what went wrong, you will be able to use reasoning to come up with a solution. Always remember to update your records and note any changes in the formula or procedure.

But if used incorrectly, reasoning can lead you astray. Many things that sound "reasonable" are actually false! It seemed reasonable to our primitive ancestors that stars were campfires and that the Earth was flat; however, we know now that this was false reasoning. Faulty reasoning is almost always based on poor observations. Many "old wives' tales" are examples of judgmental observations.

For instance, it is widely believed that long or braided hair grows faster. This belief is based on the false assumption that weight or pulling will cause hair follicles to produce keratin faster. In truth, neither has any effect on hair growth, but it sounds good. This myth was probably started by someone who thought it made sense. Be careful not to accept ideas or draw conclusions just because they sound good. Many advertisers take advantage of fallacies or myths by using fancy, "scientific" terms to fool the unsuspecting.

Use the power to reason and check with observations to find the truth, especially to analyze advertising claims. If a product is supposed to "last 50 percent longer" or "make hair feel silkier than the leading brand," test these claims and don't automatically accept them as fact.

Testing

The best way to test reasoning is by experimenting. An experiment allows a person to make good observations and draw conclusions about what was actually seen. In a sense, each time you try a new product or procedure, you are conducting an experiment. Based on the outcome of the personal evaluation, you will draw conclusions about a product's or procedure's success or failure.

Each experiment is a test of your ideas and knowledge. Every idea must be continually tested and retested. Each chemical service you perform and every change you make must be carefully observed and recorded. New information can be observed with each experiment that will test the correctness of your ideas. If we learn by our mistakes, we won't have to repeat them.

Too often, hairstylists are hesitant to try new things. It is easy to become set in one's ways, but this can hinder professional growth. A positive way to excel in the field of cosmetology is through experimentation. However, we must always consider the client's well-being and our own safety or liability. Testing products on swatches of hair is an excellent way to try a new one.

Proper experimentation with products or procedures should not be based on off-the-wall ideas or wild guesses. Clients do not appreciate this type of irresponsibility. Good experiments are based on previous observations and careful reasoning. The best ideas for experiments usually come from education and experience. Top-notch hairstylists are those who aren't afraid to experiment, but only in careful, controlled manner. Remember, the chemicals used for cosmetology services are tools and not toys! Treat them with the respect they deserve.

Cause and Effect

Although more emphasis is usually placed on the art of hairstyling, the practice of cosmetology is also a science. Science is very concerned with why things work (or don't work) and how to control them. Scientists study the causes of an event. Why something happens is very important. **Cause and effect** means that things don't just happen; there is a reason for everything. When you perform a service and get an unexpected result, attempt to solve the problem with reasoning through evaluation of the observations.

The easy answer is, "Oh, I'm having a bad day" or "Something must be wrong with your hair." Answers like this do not solve problems; they make it difficult to learn and grow. Using the scientific method with observation, reasoning, and testing provides the best road to finding the correct solution. Properly used, these three steps often remove chance or luck from professional services and replace them with understanding and expertise. The best hairstylists aren't lucky—they're knowledgeable!

EXPERIMENTS YOU SHOULD NOT PERFORM

Experimentation is fun and beneficial; however, it can create problems! Manufacturers go to great lengths to develop products that provide desirable effects. *Always* read and follow the manufacturers' instructions. It is very important to heed any warnings found on the label or in the product literature.

The wise hairstylist will check periodically for changes in directions or warnings. Manufacturers often discover improved techniques or learn new information about their products. Usually, these ideas are included in the packaging as revised instructions. Disregarding instructions can have serious consequences.

Often hairstylists will attempt to develop their own special blends by mixing together chemical products that were not specifically designed for mixing. It may seem fun and exciting, but it is not a wise practice.

Many chemicals form incompatible mixtures when blended. This means, when products are mixed, the blend could be hazardous. Some mixtures could catch fire, explode, release harmful vapors, or even cause a hairstylist or client to suffer a painful allergic reaction.

The classic example of incompatible blends is the practice of mixing chlorine bleach with ammonia products. This *deadly* combination releases gases which may kill or seriously injure people. It is best to never mix any chemical products without first checking with the manufacturer.

WHAT SCIENCE IS NOT!

We learned in the beginning of this chapter that science is the systematic study of our universe. A well-known scientific researcher, studying the growth of hair, once made the following statement about finding a cure for baldness, "If we are going to understand hair growth, we are going to do it through solid, methodical science."

Don't be impressed by such extravagant claims as *amazing new discovery, scientific breakthrough,* or *revolutionary new product.* These are advertising and marketing sales tools, not truly science. When you perform chemical services, don't depend on miracle products. Instead, trust in the scientific method, observation, reasoning, and testing. You'll be much more likely to get positive results.

Other Sources of Information

It is important to stay in touch with new information because products are constantly changing. New ideas or techniques emerge almost daily. Where can information be found to keep you on the cutting edge? Check the following:

1. Manufacturer- and distributor-sponsored educational classes. These are excellent sources for information.

2. Trade show educational classes. These are special sessions taught by the experts in the field.

3. Specialized schools that teach advanced topics; i.e., haircolor or hair-cutting seminars.

4. Trade magazines are often mostly advertisements, but if you thoroughly read through the pages, you'll often find a wealth of information on highly specialized topics.

5. Ask your instructors. If you show an interest in learning more than what the book has to offer, they will guide you to outside sources of information.

6. The appendix to this textbook.

REVIEW QUESTIONS

1. What are the three basic steps of learning in the scientific method?

2. If you noticed that your client develops a rash each time you use permanent haircolor, which of these three basic steps did you use?

3. Give two examples of something that sounds reasonable but is actually false.

4. What is the difference between cause and effect? Give an example.

5. Why is it important to periodically reread the manufacturer's instructions?

6. Name three sources where you can find information found in the book or taught in class.

DISCUSSION QUESTIONS

1. Science has radically changed our understanding of hair and skin. What futuristic products can you imagine might be developed in the next decade?

2. In what ways will scientific advancements change cosmetology? What should cosmetologists do to keep up with this new technology?

Chapter 2

The Structure of Life

Key Terms

Biology
Cells
Cell membrane
Centrosome
CHONS elements
Cytoplasm
Entropy
Nuclear membrane
Nucleoli
Nucleolus
Nucleus
Mitochondria
Mitosis
Organelles
Organic compounds
Ribosomes

Learning Objectives

After completing this chapter, you should be able to:

- Understand the difference between the terms *organic* and *inorganic*.

- What is the first rule of biology?

- Identify the inner parts of a cell.

- Describe how living cells grow and divide.

THE MIRACLE OF LIFE

Everything in the universe has a natural tendency to lose energy and become more disordered. This loss of energy is referred to as **entropy** (**EN**-troh-pee). Entropy is what happens to your bedroom if you don't make an effort to keep it clean. Entropy is also the reason your lunch spoils if you forget to put it in the refrigerator. Decay is the natural state of matter and entropy is the force that drives it.

In a universe ruled by entropy and constantly drawn toward greater disorder, the beauty and mystery of life is its ability to create an organized form from formlessness. Life organizes matter. The magic of life is its ability to draw order from a sea of disorder. All living organisms have the gift of creating order on themselves, which permits them to escape the force of entropy.

Although scientists can observe the birth of simple organic molecules, they cannot generate life from nonliving matter. George Washington Carver created more than 300 different products from peanuts but was unable to change even one of them back into a peanut.

Biology is the science of the study of living things. The word combines "bio" which means life and "ology" which means the study of. The study of biology is essential for hairstylists because it relates to hair and skin. The first rule of biology is that all forms of life need the element carbon to exist. This is true for everything that has ever lived. All plants, animals, and bacteria are made of carbon. Without this element, life as we know it would not exist. Carbon is the backbone of nature.

Carbon is only one of ninety different elements that are found in nature. Hydrogen is the lightest element and uranium is the heaviest.

Our bodies contain many other elements, but the most important is carbon. Hydrogen, oxygen, and nitrogen together account for over 78 percent of the human body. In the body, they combine with carbon (or each other) to form compounds. When elements combine to form compounds, they become molecules. Carbon combines with oxygen, hydrogen, and nitrogen to make an unlimited number of different compounds.

Chemists use shorthand abbreviations to show what elements are in a molecule. Carbon is represented by a capital C, H stands for Hydrogen, O represents Oxygen, N is for Nitrogen, and S is for Sulfur. Since these are the elements which make skin, nails, and hair, it is important to remember them and their symbols. It is easy to remember these elements of life if you arrange the symbols into a word. They become the **CHONS elements**. These elements make up more than 99 percent of the body.

Compounds that contain carbon are called **organic compounds.** Since anything that lives must contain carbon, all living things are *organic*. Skin and hair are organic matter. They are made from many large molecules of the CHONS elements. When millions of these large molecules group together into microscopic communities, they are called **cells.** Now you can see why carbon, along with other elements, are the building blocks of nature. The way these elements combine is the basis for all living things

This topic is discussed in further detail in chapter 8.

IT'S ORGANIC

One of the most misused words in the beauty industry is *organic*. Advertisers realize that the public has a misconception of this term. They have promoted its use to sell everything from vitamins to shampoo.

Most people believe that organic means that the product is healthy, safe, or natural. To some it means no artificial ingredients or preservatives are used. Still others think organic products are good for the preservation of our environment.

In truth, this word has little real meaning for the average consumer. Organic means a substance contains the element carbon in its chemical structure. Almost all artificial ingredients in foods and cosmetics are organic. Pesticides and preservatives are commonly made of organic compounds. Even smog and cigarette smoke are organic. The famous philosopher Socrates was forced by his enemies to drink hemlock, a poisonous, organic herb.

Cow manure and crude oil are organic, but most people would not want them as an ingredient in shampoo or skin cream. *Don't be fooled!* If you buy products simply because they are organic, you're probably getting less than you bargained for!

CELLS

In 1665, the English scientist Robert Hooke tried a new, more powerful type of microscope. When he looked at thin slices of cork he saw many small boxlike structures. He called them cells, from the Latin word for "chamber." The cells he saw were dead and empty. It would not be known for another two hundred years that all living things were made of cells. This word is still used today as the name for the smallest piece of organized living matter.

There are nearly ten trillion cells in your body, and every one of them came from only two original cells, a female egg cell and a male sperm cell. Cells die and are replaced at the fantastic rate of fifty million each second. In our body, cells carry food and oxygen. They also fight bacteria. Without cells we could not see, hear, or taste. Cells digest our food as well as store our thoughts and memories (Fig. 2.1).

There are three main parts to a cell.

1. The **cell membrane** (**MEM**-brayn) or **wall** encloses a single cell and separates it from other cells. It allows food in and lets waste pass out of the cell.

2. The **nucleus** (**NOO**-klee-us) is the control center of the cell. The nucleus directs the cell's activity, organizes its work, and stores reproductive genes.

3. The **cytoplasm** (**SY**-toh-plaz-em) is a clear jellylike substance that fills the cell membrane. The nucleus and other smaller bodies float in this thick fluid.

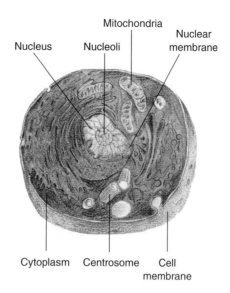

Figure 2-1 *Diagram of a typical cell.*
(Courtesy: N. Richardson)

Suspended in the cytoplasm are small bodies that the nucleus uses to perform the cell's work. These bodies are called **organelles** or little organs. Just as we have organs in our body to breathe and digest food, the same is true for cells. Cells are much like little cities.

A city needs a lot of power to run, and so do cells. One very important organelle is the **mitochondria** (migh-to-**KON**-dree-uh). These are the powerhouses of the cell. They provide the energy that cells need to do work. A cell in the muscle, for instance, may have hundreds of tiny power plants.

Nucleoli (new-**KLEE**-oh-lye) are located in a region within the nucleus. Most cells have two or more nucleoli. The nucleolus (singular) is the site of ribosomal RNA synthesis and consists of ribosomal RNA and ribosomal protein. After the ribosomes are manufactured in the nucleoli, they move through the pores in the nuclear membrane and pass into the cytoplasm.

The **nuclear membrane** is the outer boundary of the nucleus. Openings called nuclear pores are located at various spots on its surface and serve as passageways for molecules entering and leaving the nucleus.

The **centrosome** (**SEN**-tro-sohm) is a spherical region in the cytoplasm with no apparent structure. It may vary in size from one cell type to another, and although it is generally free of organelles, it may contain ribosomes and mitochondria.

Ribosomes (**RY**-bo-sohms) are the small spherical structures where proteins are manufactured.

Skin cells die quickly. Normal abrasion, sunlight, and defending against invaders are just a few reasons for quick cell turnover. Old cells that die are replaced

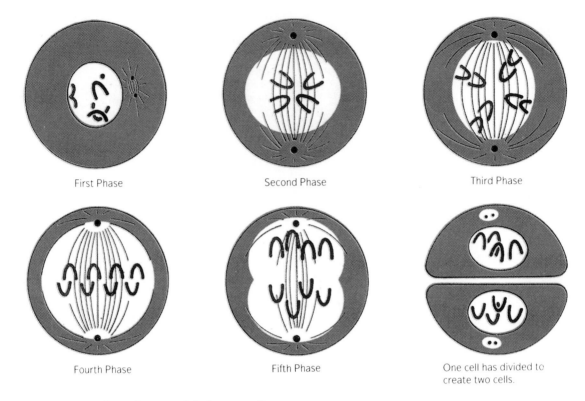

| First Phase | Second Phase | Third Phase |
| Fourth Phase | Fifth Phase | One cell has divided to create two cells. |

Figure 2-2 *Indirect division of the human cell.*
(Courtesy: CEM)

by new cells that are produced in a process of cell division called **mitosis** (migh-**TO**-sis). Although it may seem like magic, mitosis is a simple process.

The nucleus stretches and splits in half. A new cell wall forms between the two halves and forms two cells. The cells are identical. When these new cells divide again, their offspring are identical to the original cell. It is by mitosis that hair grows and skin cells are replaced (Fig. 2.2).

The epidermis is in a continual state of renewal as the cells are formed, mature, and die. The epidermis completely renews itself every forty-five to seventy-five days. Keratinocytes are formed by mitosis in the basal layer of the epidermis and move upward through the epidermis as they mature in a process called keratinization. As newly formed keratinocytes mature, they fill with keratin, move upward, flatten out, lose their nucleus and die. The cells in the outer most layer of the stratum corneum flake off and are replaced by new cells from below. It is estimated that a new cell takes twenty-eight days to reach the stratum corneum. Every day the top layer of the stratum corneum is shed, as a new replacement layer is formed, by mitosis, in the stratum granulosum below.

THE BIG PICTURE

Clients have a limited view of the hair and skin. They see only the big picture, the final results. As a hairstylist, you must be concerned with the structure of the hair and the condition of the cells.

Atoms are the basic structure and the building blocks of all matter. Atoms of different elements combine to form compounds (Chapter 8, General Chemistry), and those compounds make up all the cells of the body. The organization and structure of the body begins with its cells. Cells make up tissues, tissues make up organs, and organs make up systems. Every structure of our body can be broken down into cells and understanding those cells allows us to understand ourselves.

REVIEW QUESTIONS

1. Find the name of each element for these chemical symbols: C, H, O, N, S.

2. If a cell in your skin divided by mitosis and both cells divided again and then every cell divided again, how many new cells are formed?

3. What portion of the cell provides the energy for mitosis and other functions?

DISCUSSION QUESTIONS

1. How does the actual definition of "organic" differ from the everyday use of the word? In what way could a misconception like this be dangerous?

2. Why is it important that hairstylists understand the properties of cells?

Chapter 3

Microbiology

Key Terms

Bacilli
Bacteria
Bacteriology
Cocci
Contagious or communicable
Diplococci
Flagella or cilia
Fungi
General infection
HIV & AIDS
Immunity
Local infection
Microorganisms
Motile
Nonpathogenic
Pathogenic
Protozoa
Rickettsia
Saprophytes
Spirilla
Staphylococci
Streptococci
Viruses

Learning Objectives

After completing this chapter, you should be able to:

- List the types and classifications of bacteria.

- Understand how bacteria grow and reproduce.

- Understand the difference between pathogenic and nonpathogenic bacteria.

- Understand how contagious diseases are spread.

- Understand AIDS and how it is spread.

INTRODUCTION

There are many different types of **microorganisms** (meye-kroh-**OR**-gah-niz-ems), which are commonly referred to as microbes or germs. An understanding of how these germs grow and how they spread will help prevent both you and your client from contracting an infectious disease.

Bacteriology (bak-teer-ee-**OL**-o-jee) is the study of bacteria. *Bacteria* (bak-**TEER**-ee-ah) are the oldest, most abundant and simplest organisms on Earth. Bacteria are one-celled vegetable microorganisms that are present on and in everything you touch. They do not depend on other organisms to live and can live outside the human body. Although there are hundreds of different kinds of bacteria, they can all be classified as one of two types.

1. Nonpathogenic bacteria do not produce disease.

All bacteria do not produce disease. Many are harmless, some are helpful, and others are essential for life on Earth. Helpful bacteria are used to produce yogurt, sauerkraut, pickles, and olives. Nitrogen-fixing bacteria convert nitrogen from the atmosphere into a form that can be used by plants. Other bacteria are necessary for the decomposition of organic matter, which improves the quality of soil for farming. **Saprophytes** (**SAP**-ro-fights) are **nonpathogenic** (non-path-o-**JEN**-ik) bacteria that live on dead matter and do not produce disease.

2. Pathogenic bacteria produce disease.

All infectious disease begins when **pathogenic** (path-o-**JEN**-ik) germs enter the body. Most infectious diseases are caused by one of six types of pathogens. The most common are **bacteria** (bak-**TEER**-ee-a) and **viruses** (**VY**-rus-es). Hairstylists must practice proper disinfection and sanitation methods to protect themselves and their clients from the spread of disease in the salon.

CLASSIFICATIONS OF PATHOGENIC BACTERIA

Pathogenic bacteria cause tetanus, meningitis, scarlet fever, strep throat, tuberculosis, gonorrhea, syphilis, chlamydia, toxic shock syndrome, Legionnaires' disease, diphtheria, and food poisoning. The three main classes of pathogenic bacteria are determined by their distinctive shapes. (Fig. 3.1)

1. **Cocci** (**KOK**-si) are round-shaped organisms that appear alone or in groups. There are three groups of cocci: (Fig. 3.2)

a) **Staphylococci** (staf-i-lo-**KOK**-si) grow in bunches or clusters. They are pus-forming and cause abscesses, pustules, and boils.

b) **Streptococci** (strep-to-**KOK**-si) grow in chains. They are pus-forming and cause strep throat.

c) **Diplococci** (dip-lo-**KOK**-si) grow in pairs and cause pneumonia.

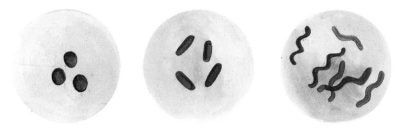

Figure 3-1 *General forms of bacteria.*

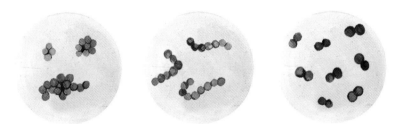

Figure 3-2 *Groupings of bacteria.*

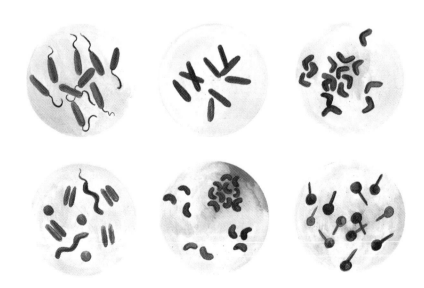

Figure 3-3 *Disease-producing bacteria.*

2. **Bacilli** (ba-**SIL**-I) are short rod-shaped organisms. They are the most common type of bacteria and cause tetanus, flu, typhoid fever, tuberculosis, and diphtheria. (Fig. 3.3)

3. **Spirilla** (sp-**RIL**-a) are spiraled organisms that cause syphilis and cholera.

MOVEMENT OF BACTERIA

Both bacilli and spirilla are **motile**, which means they have the ability to move by themselves. The whip-like motion of tiny hair-like projections, known as **flagella** (flah-**JEL**-a) or **cilia** (**SIL**-ee-a), propels bacteria through liquids. Cocci rarely show motility. They are spread through the air, in dust, and by contact with people and objects.

BACTERIAL GROWTH AND REPRODUCTION

The two distinct stages in the life cycle of bacteria are an active stage and an inactive stage.

1. **The Active or Vegetative Stage**

   Bacteria grow and reproduce during this stage. Warm, dark, damp places with sufficient food provide the most favorable conditions for rapid growth. Bacteria reproduce every one to three hours, by mitosis (see chapter 2). This rapid doubling of cells allows most bacteria to produce a population of billions in just one day.

2. **The Inactive or Spore-Forming Stage**

   In order to survive when conditions for growth are not favorable, some bacteria such as anthrax and tetanus become inactive and form spores resistant to heat and disinfectants. When favorable conditions return, the spores return to the active or vegetative stage, then grow and reproduce.

VIRUSES

Viruses (**VY**-rus-es) are much smaller than bacteria and do not have a cellular structure. Viruses depend on other organisms to live and reproduce, and unlike bacteria, viruses can't live outside of the body. Viruses are not killed or weakened by antibiotics as are bacteria. Viruses cause hepatitis, tuberculosis, measles, mumps, chicken pox, meningitis, rubella, influenza, warts, colds, herpes, shingles, genital warts, and AIDS.

The Human Immunodeficiency Virus (**HIV**) causes Acquired Immune Deficiency Syndrome (**AIDS**). HIV attacks white blood cells and destroys the body's ability to fight infection. The infections that strike people whose immune systems

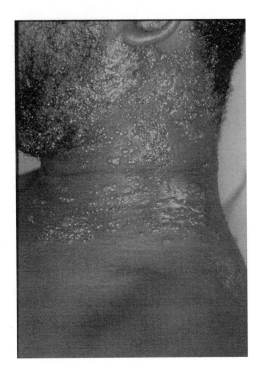

Figure 3-4 *Herpes Type II in an HIV-positive patient.*
(Courtesy Rube J. Pardo, M.D., Ph.D.)

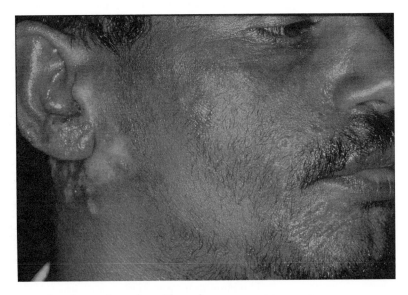

Figure 3-5 *Shingles on the neck and face of an HIV-positive patient.*
(Courtesy Rube J. Pardo, M.D., Ph. D.)

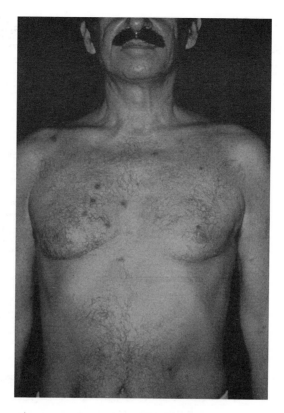

Figure 3-6 *Kaposi's sarcoma in an AIDS (HIV-positive) patient.*
(Courtesy Rube J. Pardo, M.D., Ph. D.)

are weakened by HIV include severe pneumonia and fungal infections of the mouth and esophagus. Those infected with HIV may also develop Kaposi's sarcoma and other unusual cancers.

In spite of what you may have heard, HIV cannot be spread through casual contact. HIV is only transmitted through exposure to infected blood, semen, or vaginal secretions. According to the American Red Cross, HIV is easily killed by alcohol, chlorine bleach, and other common disinfectants.

OTHER INFECTIOUS AGENTS

Fungi (FUN-ji) are plant parasites, such as molds, mildews, and yeasts that cause athlete's foot and ringworm.

Protozoa (PROH-toh-zoh-h) are animal-like organisms that cause malaria and dysentery.

Rickettsia cause typhus and Rocky Mountain spotted fever.

Animal parasites cause contagious diseases. The itch mite causes scabies and head lice cause pediculosis.

TYPES OF INFECTION

There are two types of infection.

1. A **local infection** is limited to a small, specific area and is indicated by a boil or pimple that contains pus.

2. A **general infection** is also called a *systemic infection* because the bloodstream carries the pathogens and toxins to all parts of the body.

Contagious (kon-**TAY**-jus) or **communicable** (ko-**MYOO**-ni-kah-bil) diseases are those that can be spread from one infected person to another. Infectious diseases are usually spread through contact by unclean hands, implements, and unsanitary salon conditions. Pathogens enter the body through open sores, breaks in the skin, and body openings such as the mouth, eyes, and nose.

IMMUNITY

Immunity (Im-**MYOO**-ni-tee) is the body's ability to destroy pathogens and resist disease. There are two types of immunity:

1. Natural immunity is a natural resistance to disease, which is partly inherited and the result of a healthy immune system.

2. Acquired immunity occurs after the body overcomes a disease or as a result of inoculation.

REVIEW QUESTIONS

1. What are bacteria?
2. List several diseases caused by bacteria.
3. What are viruses?
4. List several diseases caused by viruses.
5. What are pathogens?
6. How do bacteria multiply?
7. List and define the three forms of bacteria.
8. How do bacteria move about?
9. How do pathogens enter the body?

DISCUSSION QUESTIONS

1. What are microbes, microorganisms and germs?
2. How are most contagious diseases spread?
3. What can you do to prevent the spread of disease in the salon?
4. How can bacteria be destroyed?
5. How can viruses be destroyed?

Chapter 4

The Structure of Skin

Key Terms

Adipose
Carotene
Dermis
Endocrine glands
Epidermis
Erythema
Exocrine glands
Keratin
Keratinization
Mast cells
Melanin
Nerve endings
Organs
Papillary layer
Reticular layer
Sebaceous glands
Sebum
Subcutaneous
Sudoriferous glands
The Sun Protection Factor (SPF)
Tissues
Trans Epidermal Water Loss
Ultraviolet radiation

Learning Objectives

After completing this chapter, you should be able to:

- Describe each type of tissue and its specialization.

- Identify the main layers of skin and understand their differences.

- List the function of different nerves found in the skin.

- List the function of the different skin glands.

- Explain the causes and types of skin color.

- Understand the difference between UVA, UVB, and UVC.

TISSUE

There are over 100 different types of cells that form the structures of the human body. These cells are organized into tissues. **Tissues** are groups of similar cells that work together to perform a specific function. Two or more types of tissues that are grouped together to form a functional unit are called **organs**. The skin, which includes the hair and nails, is the largest organ of the human body.

Tissue is made up of large groups of cells that are similar in function. There are five types of tissue found in the body.

1. *Connective tissue* supports and protects the organs. It also holds other tissues together. Cartilage, ligaments, and tendons are examples of this type of tissue.

2. *Muscular tissue* gives the ability to move various parts of the body. Movement is caused when muscular tissues contract (shorten) or relax. Muscle tissue also protects delicate internal organs.

3. *Nerve tissue* carries instructions from the brain to the various parts of the body. Nerve tissue cells also send messages to the brain (e.g., touch and sight).

4. *Liquid tissue* carries oxygen and food to other tissue cells and also removes waste from the body. These are individual cells, not linked by connective tissue. Blood and lymph fluid are examples of liquid tissue.

5. *Epithelial* (ep-i-**THEEL**-ee-ul) *tissue* gives a protective covering to the body and internal organs. Skin is epithelial tissue, as is the lining of the stomach, heart, and lungs. This type of tissue repairs itself very quickly.

Each different type of tissue is made of cells designed to perform a special job. This is called *specialization*. Examples of specialization are seen everywhere in the body. Cells inside the eye are very good at seeing colors but would not work well as muscle cells. Few parts of the body have as many different specialized cells as the skin (Figs. 4-1–4-5)

SKIN

The skin is a thick, tough layer of tissue cells that surrounds the body. Skin acts as a barrier to keep out harmful bacteria, fungi, and viruses. It is the largest body organ in size (three thousand square inches!), but weighs only six pounds. Skin consists of many layers and types of specialized cells as shown in Figures 4-6 and 4-7.

Skin has three main layers:

1. **epidermis** (ep-e-**DUR**-mis), the outermost layer.
2. **dermis** (**DUR**-mis), the middle layer.
3. **subcutaneous** (sub-cue-**TAY**-nee-us) **tissue**, the deepest layer.

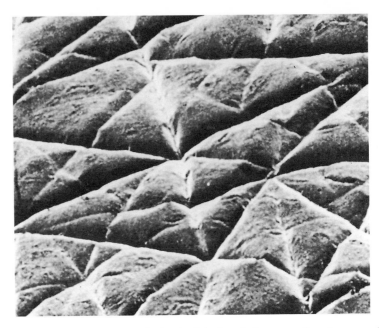

Figure 4-1 *Photo of the skin on the back of the hand of a young female, magnified 60 times. Notice the triangular appearance of the major divisions of the skin surface.*
(Courtesy: Gillette Company Research Institute, Rockville, Maryland)

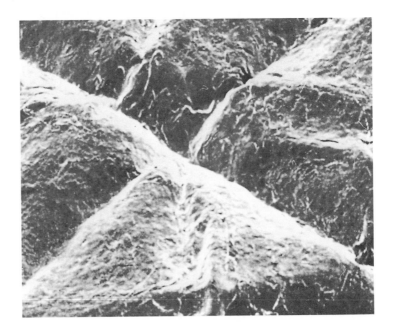

Figure 4-2 *The same skin section magnified 176 times. Notice the edges of the individual stratum corneum cells adhering tightly to the skin.*
(Courtesy: Gillette Company Research Institute, Rockville, Maryland)

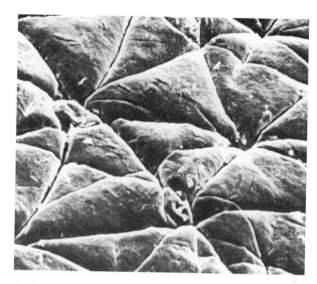

Figure 4-3 *Cheek of a young female, magnified 210 times. Notice that the surface looks more plump and more rounded than the back of the hand photos. This probably is the result of more moisture in the skin. Follicle openings can be seen in the center of the photo.*
(Courtesy: Gillette Company Research Institute, Rockville, Maryland)

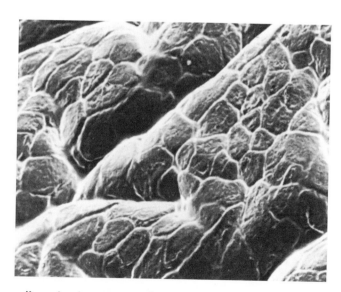

Figure 4-4 *Elbow skin from a young female, magnified 60 times. Notice how the overall architecture of the skin differs from previous skin photos. This indicates that skin from different areas has very different structures.*
(Courtesy: Gillette Company Research Institute, Rockville, Maryland)

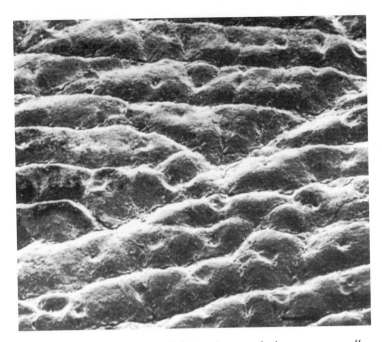

Figure 4-5 *The skin from the palm of the hand, magnified 60 times. Small indentations of ridges are sweat gland openings.*
(Courtesy: Gillette Research Institute, Rockville, Maryland)

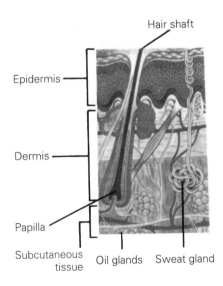

Hair shaft

Epidermis

Dermis

Papilla

Subcutaneous tissue

Oil glands

Sweat gland

Figure 4-6 *Microscopic section of new skin.*

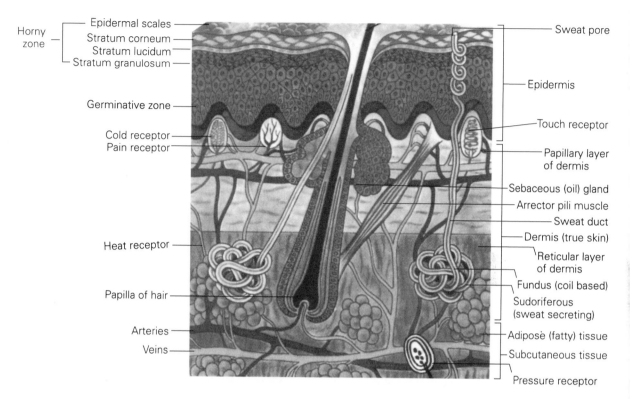

Horny zone
- Epidermal scales
- Stratum corneum
- Stratum lucidum
- Stratum granulosum

Germinative zone

Cold receptor
Pain receptor

Heat receptor

Papilla of hair

Arteries

Veins

Sweat pore

Epidermis

Touch receptor

Papillary layer of dermis

Sebaceous (oil) gland

Arrector pili muscle

Sweat duct

Dermis (true skin)

Reticular layer of dermis

Fundus (coil based)

Sudoriferous (sweat secreting)

Adiposè (fatty) tissue

Subcutaneous tissue

Pressure receptor

Figure 4-7 *Cross section of the skin.*

Subcutaneous Tissue

Subcutaneous tissue consists mainly of connective tissue, blood veins and arteries, lymph fluid vessels, fat cells, hair papilla, and sensitive nerve endings. Arteries in the subcutaneous tissue supply the upper levels of the skin with food and oxygen.

Veins carry carbon dioxide and waste away from the cells. Since blood vessels do not enter the epidermis, oxygen and nutrients must be fed to the cells from the blood vessels in the subcutaneous layer.

Adipose (AD-I-poce), or **fat tissue,** is found in the subcutaneous layer. It helps give the body smooth curves and contours. Adipose tissue accounts for about 14 percent of the average person's body weight. The fat cells cushion the internal organs from bumps and bangs and can be used for energy. Adipose tissue also helps to insulate the body from extreme cold or heat.

Dermis Tissue

The *dermis* (**DUR**-mis) is the middle layer of skin, located directly above the subcutaneous tissue and below the epidermis.

The dermis layer makes up 90 percent of the skin's dry weight. This tissue collects nutrients from the subcutaneous layer and passes them to the upper layers. In some body locations, like the eyelid, the dermis is very thin. It is several times thicker on the soles of the feet and palms of the hands. This skin layer is made mostly of protein fibers and specialized types of cells.

The strong protein fibers of the dermis are connective tissue. They penetrate into the subcutaneous tissue, tightly bonding the two layers together. The dermis is made up of two layers: the papillary, or superficial layer, and the reticular or deeper layer. The **papillary** (pah-**PIL**-ah-ry) **layer** is the upper layer of the dermis and lies directly below the epidermis. It contains *papillae* (pah-**PIL**-ee), *capillaries* (**KAP**-ih-ler-ees), and *tactile corpuscles* (**TAK**-til **KOR**-pus-els). The lower part of the dermis is called the **reticular layer.** In this layer the protein fibers finely interlace into netlike patterns. Hair follicles grow between spaces in this net. These fibers are made of two types of protein, *collagen* and *elastin*.

Collagen comes from the Greek word meaning "to produce glue." Animal collagen has been used for thousands of years to make strong glues, such as white paper glue. In humans, it makes up about 75 percent of the skin's dry weight. Collagen is to the skin as the frame is to a house or car; it gives strength and support.

Elastin is a unique and very different skin protein. It accounts for only 2 percent of the skin's dry weight, but is still very important. Elastin is much like a rubber band. It can be stretched to twice its length and still bounce back to its original size and shape; likewise, elastin gives skin the ability to stretch while keeping its shape. It acts like the shock absorbers on a car. As skin ages, it contains less elastin, thus becoming less elastic.

Mast cells go unnoticed in the skin until damage occurs. When the skin is cut, burned, or chemically irritated, these unique cells spring into action. First, mast cells release a chemical that stops bleeding. Later, mast cells increase the flow of blood to the injury, thus speeding the healing process. Mast cells also cause redness and swelling in skin after burns or allergic reactions.

Epidermis Tissue

Epidermis tissue is the uppermost layer of skin. The purpose of the epidermal cells is to make the skin resistant to water and to prevent invasion from outside the body (Figs. 4-8 and 4-9). The epidermis is only about fifty cell layers thick and is twenty-five times thinner than the dermis. The epidermis is divided into four layers or *strata* (**STRAT**-uh):

1. *Stratum germinativum* (jur-mi-nah-**TIV**-um) is the basement of the epidermis. It is only one cell layer thick, but from here the rest of the

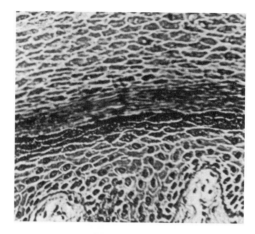

Figure 4-8 *Section of skin showing thickened epidermis on the sole of the foot.*

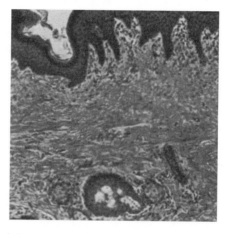

Figure 4-9 *Section of skin showing thinner epidermis on the back of the hand.*

epidermis "germinates" or grows. This single row of cells constantly undergoes mitosis, each cell dividing into two. As these cells multiply, they are pushed toward the surface. This is the beginning of a long, upward journey which eventually brings the cell to the surface of the skin. As these cells are pushed upward, they undergo a remarkable change.

2. *Stratum granulosum* (gran-yoo-**LOH**-sum) layer contains cells that have become flat and hard. This is the first step in **keratin** formation. Keratin is the water-resistant protein found in the upper layers of the epidermis.

The importance of keratin will be discussed in later chapters. In this stratum, the cells begin to die as their nuclei break down.

3. *Stratum lucidum* (**LOO**-si-dum) is completely transparent to light. These cells no longer contain a nucleus.

4. *Stratum corneum* (**KOHR**-nee-um) is about thirty rows thick. The cells in this layer look little like they did in the stratum germinativum. They no longer contain organelles and are completely filled with keratin. The stratum corneum is the barrier that repels heat waves, light, bacteria, and some chemicals. It is important to remember, however, that this barrier is not impenetrable. Many types of chemicals, safe and harmful, can rapidly penetrate this extremely thin cell shield.

As these mature cells reach the surface of the skin, they are continually being shed. In this way, the upper layers of the skin's surface are constantly replaced by cells born in the stratum germinativum.

The epidermis is in a continual state of renewal as the cells are formed, mature, and die. The epidermis completely renews itself every 45 to 75 days. Keratinocytes are formed by mitosis in the basal layer of the epidermis and move upward through the epidermis as they mature in a process called **keratinization**. As newly formed keratinocytes mature, they fill with keratin, move upward, flatten out, lose their nucleus, and die. The cells in the outer most layer of the stratum corneum flake off and are replaced by new cells from below. It is estimated that a new cell takes 28 days to reach the stratum corneum. Every day, the top layer of the stratum corneum is shed as a new replacement layer is formed, by mitosis, in the stratum granulosum below.

SKIN AS A BARRIER

People are often shocked to learn that many harmful chemicals can rapidly penetrate through the skin's pores and enter the bloodstream. In fact, certain chemicals found in professional products can pass through the skin in seconds. For example, hair dyes leave obvious stains. The stain is caused when chemicals become trapped in the cells. However, some of the chemical product may not be trapped and will pass into the blood vessels of the subcutaneous layer.

In most cases, a potentially harmful chemical must first enter your body before it can become a danger. If you keep it off your skin, it can't harm you! Read product labels and instructions. If the manufacturer warns against skin contact, wear gloves and wash your hands after each use!

Prolonged or repeated contact with certain products can have risks ranging from skin rash to long-term health problems. Protect yourself and work wisely to avoid unnecessary problems.

Nerve Endings

The skin contains about one million **nerve endings**. Nerve fibers transmit information from their sensitive ends through the spinal cord instantly to the brain. Nerve endings can pick up a variety of complex sensations. Most of the nerve endings are found in the face, arms, and legs. Only a few are found on the back. They are located on the shoulders and down the sides. Most nerve endings are found in the dermis or upper layers of subcutaneous tissue. Three major kinds of nerves are found in the skin:

1. *Sensory nerves*, which react to sensations such as heat or pressure.

2. *Secretory nerves*, which control the glands of the skin.

3. *Motor nerves*, which cause "gooseflesh" or make the hair shaft "stand on end."

There are several types of *sensory nerve endings*. Each registers a different type of sensation (Fig. 4-10). Some may even transmit more than one type of stimulation. These nerves are sensitive to the following:

- touch

- pressure

- heat

- cold

Pain sensors pick up each of the sensations but only if the stimulation is strong enough. For example, sensory nerve endings make the heat of a blow dryer feel warm on the scalp. However, if you move it too close to the scalp, the temperature

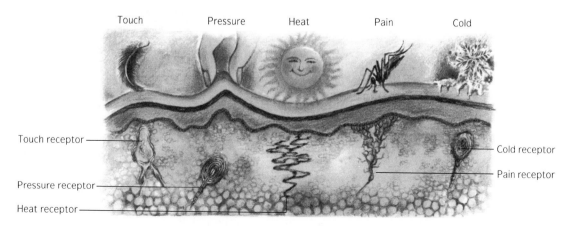

Figure 4-10 *Sensory nerves of the skin.*

skyrockets and triggers the *pain nerve endings*. They send warning messages to the brain that prevent the skin from being harmed. Sensory nerve endings show there is a lot of truth to the phrase, "There's a fine line between pleasure and pain" (Figs. 4-11 and 4-12).

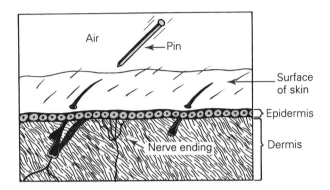

Figure 4-11 *Nerve in skin (non-active).*

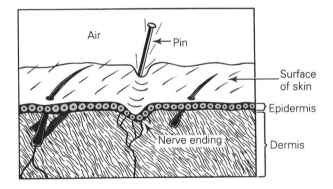

Figure 4-12 *Nerve stimulated to warn brain of injury.*

EXOCRINE GLANDS

Exocrine (**EK**-suh-krin), or duct **glands**, have canals that lead from the gland to a particular part of the body. There are two exocrine glands in the skin: the **sudoriferous** (soo-dur-**IF**-ur-us) or sweat glands, and the **sebaceous** (se-**BAY**-shus) or oil glands.

Secretory nerves control the **sudoriferous** (soo-dur-**IF**-ur-us) **(sweat) glands** (Fig. 4-13). Some parts of the skin have more than 1,300 sweat glands per square inch. The purpose of these glands is to help the body control its temperature. The sweat glands on the palms and soles also increase the "grip" of the skin

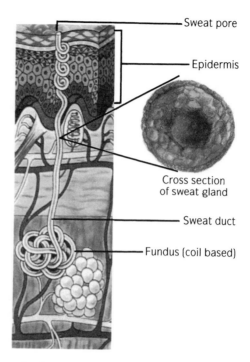

Sweat pore

Epidermis

Cross section
of sweat gland

Sweat duct

Fundus (coil based)

Figure 4-13 *Sweat gland.*

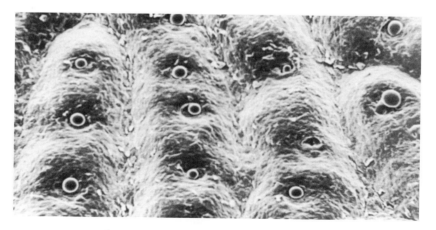

Figure 4-14 *Sweat from pores on palm of hand.*
(Courtesy: Isleworth Laboratory, Unilever Limited, Middlesex, England)

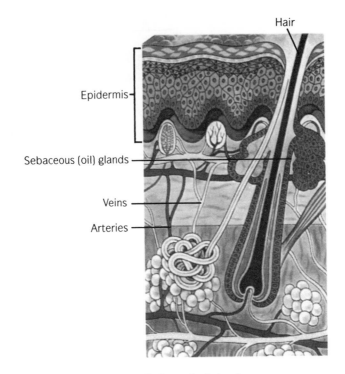

Figure 4-15 *Scalp hair, follicle, and oil glands.*

(Fig. 4-14). Evaporation of sweat has a cooling effect on the body. Sweat usually evaporates quickly, except in the armpits, which is why this area is usually moist. Sweat is odorless when it reaches the skin through the *sweat duct;* however, bacterial action on the sweat produces an offensive "sweaty" odor.

Sebaceous (se-**BAY**-shus) **(oil) glands** are also controlled by the secretory nerves (Fig. 4-15). Usually these glands are found with hair follicles. Great numbers of these oil glands are found on the scalp, face, and upper chest area but never on the soles or palms. The scalp contains as many as 1,900 glands per square inch. Sebaceous glands secrete **sebum** to the hair and skin. *Sebum* is an oily mixture of fatty substances called triglycerides along with various waxes. Many believe that sebum's function is to condition the skin and hair. It also helps the skin to retain moisture (Figs. 4-16 and 4-17).

Because *sebum* is essentially a mixture of natural oils, it reduces friction on the skin and hair. Smoothness and slipperiness of normal skin are due to the oils that coat it. There is no need to be reminded of how rough our hands can feel when the sebum has been removed by constant washing in strong soaps and detergents. The hairstylist should be aware of the role the sebum plays in preserving the natural attractiveness, as well as the essential features, of the skin.

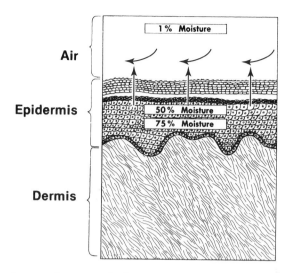

1% Moisture

Air

Epidermis

50% Moisture
75% Moisture

Dermis

Figure 4-16 *The main function of sebum is to act as a shield that prevents moisture from evaporating from the surface of the skin.*

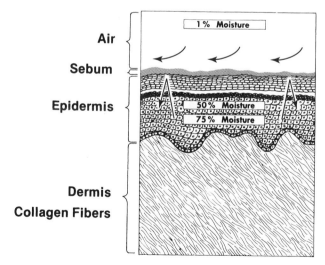

1% Moisture

Air

Sebum

Epidermis

50% Moisture
75% Moisture

Dermis
Collagen Fibers

Figure 4-17 *Summer increases the rate of sweating, and this enables the skin to stay naturally moist, preventing drying and chafing.*

Natural oils supply this external lubrication, but more important, internal lubrication is supplied by the normal moisture content of hair and skin.

Most dry skin is a result of damage to the protective layer of lipids and the *Natural Moisturizing Factor* (NMF) within the dermis. The NMF is a mixture of amino acids and salts, such as pyrrolidone carboxylic acid and lactic acid. More than half of our outer skin and about one-tenth of hair consists of water. The dry atmosphere around us poses a constant threat to the maintenance of this high lever of water. The loss of water from the internal structure of the skin to the atmosphere is referred to as **Trans Epidermal Water Loss** (TEWL). Because of the high volume of water in the cells of the skin, when we do lose moisture (for various reasons) the skin shrinks and contracts. This contraction of drying skin can break small blood vessels and cause painful pressure on nerve endings. Dry skin with cracks can easily become infected with bacteria and fungi.

Sebum also possesses powerful bacteria and fungi inhibitors that prevent the mass invasion of the skin and hair by these destructive organisms. When we consider that every object the skin touches provides more chance of attack from hostile bacteria and fungi, we realize just how much we depend on sebum for our survival. The skin would otherwise provide an ideal home for these tiny intruders, as it is warm, moist, and supplied with ample nourishment.

ENDOCRINE GLANDS

Endocrine (**EN**-duh-krin) **glands** are ductless glands that secrete hormones directly into the bloodstream, which influence the welfare of the entire body.

Skin Color

Human skin can have a surprisingly wide range of colors. Skin can be black, ghost white, red, pink, yellow, brown, olive, and dozens of different shades in between. Three factors determine the color of the skin: the pigment **melanin** (**MEL**-uh-nin), the pigment **carotene** (**KAR**-o-teen), and the blood in the capillaries of the dermis.

1. **Melanin** (**MEL**-uh-nin) is the dark pigment, which gives the skin its brown color and protects it from ultraviolet radiation. Melanin is found chiefly in the stratum germinativum of the epidermis and is contained in organelles called melanosomes. The amino acids tyrosine and cysteine are involved in melanin formation.

Depending upon the amount and type of melanin, skin can range from the palest yellow to the darkest black. An albino is a person whose skin and hair contains no melanin. The result is extremely pale white skin and hair. Sometimes, large pools of melanin collect in the skin and form freckles. Melanin protects sensitive cells from sunburn and tanning beds with ultraviolet rays. An appropriate Sun Protection Factor (SPF) lotion should be used to help the melanin in the skin protect it from burning (Figs. 4-18 and 4-19).

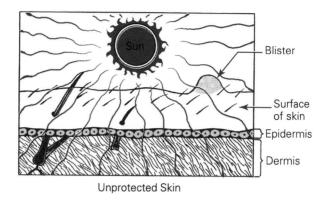

Figure 4-18 *Skin unprotected from the sun's rays.*

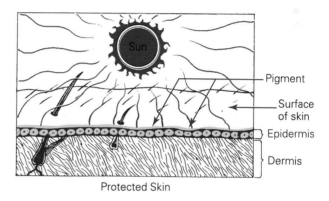

Figure 4-19 *Skin protected from the sun's rays.*

It is also possible for the skin to look blue in color, due to an optical distortion, if melanin is present at lower levels in the skin.

   2. Carotene (KAR-o-teen) is the pigment that gives yellow skin tones. Carotene is found in the stratum corneum and in the layer of fat just below the skin.

Carotene is similar to the chemical that gives carrots their color. People of Asian origin have higher amounts of carotene in their skin, which accounts for much of the yellowish hue.

   3. Blood in the small capillaries located between the dermis and the epidermis and are easily visible and add pink and red tones to the skin. Blushing occurs when these tiny vessels expand and bring the blood closer to the surface. Birthmarks are usually caused in the same way.

ULTRAVIOLET RADIATION AND SUNSCREENS

Over one million new cases of skin cancer are diagnosed each year. It is estimated that one in five Americans will develop skin cancer and 90 percent of those cancers will be the result of exposure to **ultraviolet** (UV) **radiation** from the sun and tanning beds. UV rays penetrate into the dermis and generate free radicals that can alter our DNA, the genetic material of all living cells.

In reasonable amounts, exposure to the sun is beneficial. Natural sunlight has a germicidal effect and produces vitamin D in the skin. UV radiation can be used to treat rickets, psoriasis, and acne. Exposure to UV rays also stimulates the skin's production of melanin, which causes a tan and helps protect the skin from further damage. But deep tanning is another matter, and although a deep tan may look healthy, it is really a sign that the skin is under attack from UV radiation.

Erythema (er-uh-**THEE**-muh), or redness of the skin is an inflammatory response, which appears within six hours of exposure to UV rays. The degree of redness is an indication of the amount of damage done to the skin. With each blistering sunburn, the chance of developing skin cancer is increased by 10 percent. Smoking also increases UV damage because of the formaldehyde produced in cigarette smoke.

Sunlight is a part of the electromagnetic spectrum (Fig. 4-20). *Sunlight* is made up of varying wavelengths of *electromagnetic radiation*. About 35 percent is visible light, 60 percent is *infrared radiation*, and 5 percent is made up of UV rays. UV wavelengths range from 200nm to 400nm and are further divided as follows:

UVC rays (from 200-290 nm) are the most energetic, but are the least penetrating. UVC rays are not a concern because most UVC radiation is blocked by ozone in the atmosphere and never reaches the earth.

UVB rays (from 290-320nm) are often referred to as the burning rays and are the UV radiation wavelengths most responsible for causing erythema and tanning. Erythema is used to measure the effectiveness of sunscreens and indicate the sunscreen's ability to block UVB rays. This measurement is known as the **Sun Protection Factor (SPF)**.

An SPF 2 blocks 50 percent of UVB rays, which allows you to stay in the sun twice as long as you would be able to without any protection. Increasing the SPF increases the protection. An SPF 15 blocks 93.3 percent of UVB and an SPF of 30 blocks 96.9 percent of UVB. But notice that doubling the SPF does not double the protection. In this case, it only increases UVB protection by 3.6 percent; at higher SPFs, the increase is even less. Although doubling the SPF doesn't double the protection, it does greatly increase the potential for sensitivity due to the increase in the concentration of active ingredients. UVB sunscreens include: ethylhexyl methoxycinnamate, octylsalicylate, octylhomosalate, oxybenzone, and titanium dioxide.

UVA rays (from 320-400nm) are the longest wavelengths of ultraviolet radiation and the closest to visible light. UVA is commonly known as "black light." UVA plays only a minor role in erythema and tanning, so although its affects may not be as obvious or acute as UVB, UVA exposure is every bit as damaging. UVA

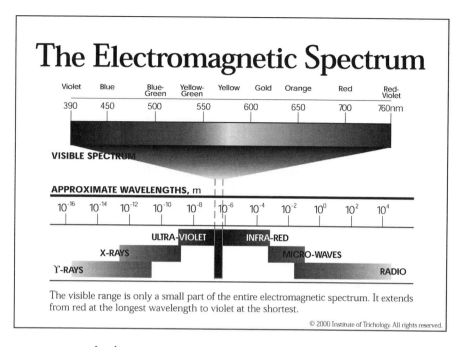

The Electromagnetic Spectrum

Violet	Blue	Blue-Green	Yellow-Green	Yellow	Gold	Orange	Red	Red-Violet
390	450	500	550	600	650	700	760nm

VISIBLE SPECTRUM

APPROXIMATE WAVELENGTHS, m

$$10^{-16} \quad 10^{-14} \quad 10^{-12} \quad 10^{-10} \quad 10^{-8} \quad 10^{-6} \quad 10^{-4} \quad 10^{-2} \quad 10^{0} \quad 10^{2} \quad 10^{4}$$

ULTRA-VIOLET   INFRA-RED

X-RAYS   MICRO-WAVES

Υ-RAYS   RADIO

The visible range is only a small part of the entire electromagnetic spectrum. It extends from red at the longest wavelength to violet at the shortest.

Figure 4-20 *The electromagnetic spectrum.*
(Reprinted with permission of Tri, Institute of Trichology)

wavelengths are the least energetic, but penetrate the deepest. Since UVA penetrates into the dermis, it contributes substantially to chronic sun damage.

Remember that SPFs only indicate protection from UVB rays and do not indicate protection from UVA rays. A sunscreen with a high SPF may provide adequate protection from UVB rays but offer little or no protection from UVA exposure. Make sure the sunscreen you use contains both UVB and UVA protection. Approved UVA sunscreens include: avobenzone (av-oh-Ben-zohn), benzophenone-3 (ben-zo-FEE-nohn), oxybenzone (ok-si-BEN-zohn), octocrylene (ok-tow-KRY-leen), menthyl anthranilate (men-thal an-thra-NY-layt), butyl methoxydibenzoylmethane (BYOO-til meth-ok-si-dy-BEN-zohl-methayn), and zinc oxide (zink OK-syd).

Many sun protection products now claim to use non-chemical sunscreens like titanium dioxide and zinc oxide. Although these inorganic sunscreens are still chemicals, they protect by physically reflecting UV rays. Traditional organic sunscreens protect by chemically absorbing UV rays. Inorganic sunscreens decrease the potential for skin irritation and sensitivity that can be caused by organic sunscreens, especially at the high concentrations required for higher SPFs. There is also some concern about unwanted chemical reactions that may take place on the skin when organic sunscreens absorb UV rays.

Although UV radiation is often referred to as UV light, UV rays are above the visible spectrum of light. UV radiation is invisible and not really light at all.

Since you can't see the UV rays that cause sunburn, it's advisable to protect yourself from the sun even on cloudy days. Although clouds block visible light, they offer little protection from damaging UV rays.

Self-tanning products make it possible to tan safely without the sun. Self-tanners contain the ingredient dihydroxyacetone (dy-hy-drohks-ee-**ASS**-ah-tohn) that reacts with the proteins on the skin's surface to turn them golden brown and simulate a natural tan.

In order to clear up the confusion about sunscreen products, the Food & Drug Administration (FDA) issued a final ruling regulating the manufacture and labeling of sunscreen products. All sunscreen products must comply with the ruling by January 1, 2003.

1. Although everyone is concerned with both UVB and UVA protection, there is currently no acceptable definition of the term "Broad Spectrum" and no standard test for UVA protection.

2. Consumers who want maximum sun protection often purchase the product with the highest SPF. Most are not aware that SPFs over 30 provide little added protection and greatly increase the dangers associated with such high concentrations of active sunscreen ingredients. The maximum SPF claim allowed on the product label will be SPF30 or SPF30 plus. For maximum protection, apply sunscreen 20 minutes before going out. Apply evenly and generously and reapply every hour.

3. Since there is no official definition of the term "natural" and all sunscreen products contain chemicals, and terms "natural," "non-chemical," and "chemical free" are considered false and misleading and are not approved. Titanium dioxide and zinc oxide are inorganic chemicals.

4. Because all sunscreens allow some UV rays to penetrate the skin, the term "sunblock" is not approved.

REVIEW QUESTIONS

1. From where does the skin receive its nourishment?
2. What keeps the dermis from pulling away from the subcutaneous layer?
3. What are the three major parts of the skin?
4. Which protein gives the skin its strength and structure?
5. Which protein gives skin elasticity?
6. Why are mast cells important?
7. Keratin is first formed in which part of the skin?
8. How does a cell in the stratum corneum differ from a cell found in the stratum germinativium?

9. What is the purpose of the sebaceous glands? The sudoriferous gland?

10. What three factors determine a person's skin color?

Discussion Questions

1. If epidermal cells are constantly rising to the surface of the skin and flaking off, why don't scars just "grow" out of the skin?

Chapter 5

Understanding Skin Disease

Key Terms

Acute cases
Allergic contact dermatitis
Chronic cases
Dermatitis
Formal Dehyde
Fungal infections
Infection
Irritant contact dermatitis
Lice
Nits
Parasites
Sarcoptes scabei
Scabies
Sensitization
Viral infections

Learning Objectives

After completing this chapter, you should be able to:

- Describe the different types of skin diseases and their causes.

- Understand the difference between an irritant reaction and an allergic reaction.

- List the causes for salon product allergy.

- Describe the different types of gloves.

- List the ways to avoid skin disease.

RECOGNIZING SKIN DISEASE

During your career as a hairstylist you will undoubtedly come in contact with skin and scalp diseases. In order to protect your own health and the health of the public, it is essential that you learn to recognize some of the more common skin diseases and know what you can and cannot do about them. A client with an inflamed skin disorder, infectious or not, should not be served in a salon. Hairstylists must be able to recognize these conditions and suggest the proper measures that need to be taken.

WHY DO HAIRSTYLISTS HAVE SKIN PROBLEMS?

Skin diseases, especially on the hands, affect one in five hairstylists. Problems relating to the skin are common in many occupations. In fact, skin disorders are the number one occupation-related disease in America.

Many chemicals produce symptoms ranging from itchy rashes to serious burns or allergies. In the salon, these problems are usually seen on the fingers, hands, wrists, and scalp.

Skin diseases and allergies force some hairstylists to give up successful careers. It is vital that hairstylists protect their hands from skin problems.

CONTACT DERMATITIS

Dermatitis (dur-muh-**TY**-tis) means an inflammation of the skin. There are two different types of contact dermatitis that are common among hairstylists:

Irritant Contact Dermatitis

Irritant Contact Dermatitis is caused by overexposure to harsh, caustic, irritating chemicals that can damage both the epidermis and dermis and cause inflammation of the tissue. Many hairstylists develop irritant contact dermatitis after years of frequent, repeated exposure to caustic and irritating salon chemicals. Irritant reactions affect everyone who comes in contact with an irritant, although the degree of irritation will vary depending on the individual. In **acute cases**, symptoms are noticed immediately or within a few hours. **Chronic cases** may take weeks, months, or years to develop. Symptoms range from redness, swelling, scaling, and itching to serious, painful chemical burns.

Extremely strong, corrosive chemicals can cause immediate, acute, and sometimes irreversible skin damage. Bleach, powdered off-the scalp hair lighteners, hydrogen peroxide, permanent wave solutions, chemical hair relaxers, and chemical depilatories are examples of corrosive salon chemicals. Serious injuries must be treated immediately by a physician.

Frequent, repeated exposure to less caustic irritants, often produces chronic contact dermatitis that can be every bit as painful as the acute form. You may find it surprising that even water, especially hard tap water, is a common salon irritant. Repeated exposure to water dries the skin. Always dry your hands completely because excessive moisture between the fingers can lead to cracking, irritation, and infection.

Frequent shampooing and hand washing also damages the skin. Hairstylists who do an excessive amount of shampooing run the greatest risk of developing chronic contact dermatitis. The harsh detergents found in many shampoos disrupt

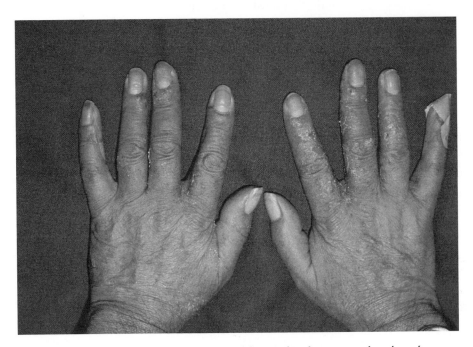

Figure 5-1   *Allergic contact dermatitis in a hairstylist due to parapheneline-diamine.*

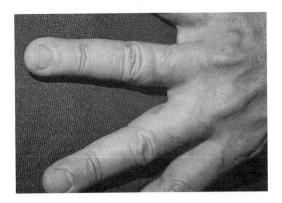

Figure 5-2   *Allergic contact dermatitis due to nickel allergy.*
(Courtesy Rube J. Pardo, M.D., Ph.D.)

YUCK! YOU'VE GOT DANDRUFF

Millions of dollars are spent each year to combat dry, flaky skin. The answer to most of these problems isn't found in a jar of expensive skin cream or medicated shampoo; the best solution is to avoid damaging the skin to begin with.

All shampoo contain detergents (surfactants) which strip away natural skin oils. Even mild shampoos must be able to dissolve oil or they're worthless. When a client sees flakes the normal reaction is to wash the hair more often. They don't realize that dandruff is usually caused by overshampooing or not thoroughly rinsing the hair.

Residual shampoo or constant washing causes prolonged and repeated exposure to irritating surfactants. The better a shampoo cleans the hair, the more likely it is that excessive use will cause dermatitis. Leaving the hair or scalp wet for long time periods can also cause itchy, dry, and flaking skin. Excessive use of hair conditioners can create problems, as well. Don't make the mistake of thinking more is better.

Prevention is the best solution. Avoid prolonged or repeated skin contact with shampoos and conditioners. Take time to rinse the hair completely and dry it thoroughly. In most cases, the dandruff will disappear on its own. However, if a skin disorder persists, recommend a dermatologist.

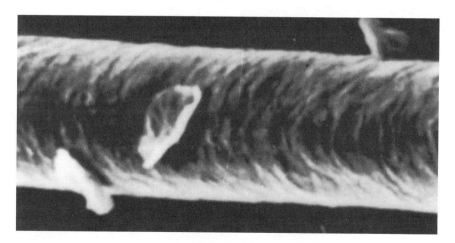

Figure 5-3 *Normal hair with dandruff flakes adhering to hair fibers.*
(Courtesy: Gillette Company Research Institute, Rockville, Maryland)

the skin's natural acid mantle, damage the protective layer of lipids (oils) and deplete the Natural Moisturizing Factor (NMF). The NMF is composed of a mixture of amino acids and salts (e.g., pyrrolidone carboxylic acid and lactic acid) which protect the skin from damage. The lipids within the epidermis also help to maintain moisture and are essential to healthy skin.

Allergic Contact Dermatitis

Normally the immune system protects us from pathogens and disease, but in the case of an allergic reaction the immune system actually causes the problem by doing its job too well. An allergic reaction occurs when our immune system mistakes a harmless substance for a toxic one and mounts a major defense. Severe allergic reactions can result in high fever and *anaphylactic* (an-ah-fah-**LAK**-tik) *shock*, which can be life threatening.

An allergic reaction is an immune system response that is caused by repeated exposure to an allergen (sensitizer). Initial exposure to an allergen will not cause an allergic reaction. The development of hypersensitivity is the result of repeated exposure to an allergen over time. This process is called **sensitization** (**SEN**-sih-tiz-a-shun) and may take months or years depending on the allergen and the intensity of exposure.

That's why the FDA requires that a patch test be performed 24–48 hours prior to each application of any aniline dye. Although your client may not have a reaction the first few times you apply the color, sensitivity may still develop after continued exposure. Although you may have colored a client's hair repeatedly in the past without an allergic reaction, that's no guarantee that your same client won't experience an allergic reaction with the next application, even with the same formula. A patch test, prior to each color application, is the only way to know if your client has become sensitized and is prone to an allergic reaction.

Poison ivy is a common allergen. Although approximately 75 percent of the population is allergic to poison ivy, the remaining 25 percent will never have a reaction no matter how many times they are exposed. Individuals who are not predisposed never become sensitized and won't develop allergies. Also remember

ARE YOU ALLERGIC TO SCISSORS?

Many hairstylists with allergic contact dermatitis are actually sensitive to their scissors. Nickel-plated scissors, pins, clips, rods, and rollers are believed to be the third leading cause of allergic reactions.

Nickel is one of the most common contact allergens in the world. Studies show that 11 percent of people tested are sensitive to nickel. Usually, nickel-plated jewelry and earrings are to blame. One study revealed that young girls with pierced ears are ten times more likely to be allergic to nickel.

If you have pierced ears, there is a good chance that you are already sensitized to nickel. Skin contact with this metal can cause dermatitis in the sensitive individual.

If you develop a rash or irritation where the scissors touch the skin, switch to a brand that is not nickel-plated. If the skin problem doesn't go away, see a dermatologist for treatment.

that different people develop allergies to different allergens. Individual predisposition may be inherited, as sensitivity seems to run in families.

The symptoms of allergic reactions are similar to those caused by simple irritants. Previously irritated, broken, or damaged skin increases the chance of developing an allergy. Unlike irritant contact dermatitis, the symptoms are not always isolated to the contact area. Swelling and other signs may occur far from the point of contact, and symptoms may take as long as 48 hours to appear. The most common culprits of **allergic contact dermatitis** are semi-permanent and permanent (oxidation) haircoloring products.

Formaldehyde (for-**MAL**-duh-hyd) is also commonly know as formalin, paraformaldehyde, oxymethylene, formic aldehyde, or methanal. Formaldehyde is a biocide that is used in cosmetics as a preservative. Formaldehyde is toxic by inhalation, a strong irritant, and a carcinogen. Formaldehyde is a sensitizer that may cause allergic reactions, even at low concentrations.

Skin Infection

Infection (in-**FEK**-shun) occurs when pathogenic microorganisms gain access to the body, overcome the body's natural defenses, multiply, and cause injury. The four groups of pathogens that cause infection are bacteria, fungi, parasites, and viruses.

Bacterial Infection

Approximately 80 percent of teenagers experience acne. Acne is a common, complex, and chronic disease that is caused by the blockage of hair follicles. The characteristic blackheads and whiteheads are called comedones. Fortunately for most people, acne usually clears up by itself once they reach their early twenties. Acne is the most common *bacterial infection*.

Fungal Infections

Fungi live on the skin and are harmless when in balance with "normal" bacteria. **Fungal infections** usually develop after these "normal" bacteria have been killed by treatment with antibiotics. Tinea pedis, commonly known as athlete's foot, is the most common fungal infection.

Parasitic Infections

The skin can become infested with **parasites**. **Scabies** is caused when the mite **Sarcoptes scabei** buries into the skin and lays eggs, leading to itching and inflammation. **Lice** are flat, wingless insects that attach to the body and suck blood. Their eggs, which attach to the hair, are called **nits**. Treatments for these infestations are available as over the counter drugs.

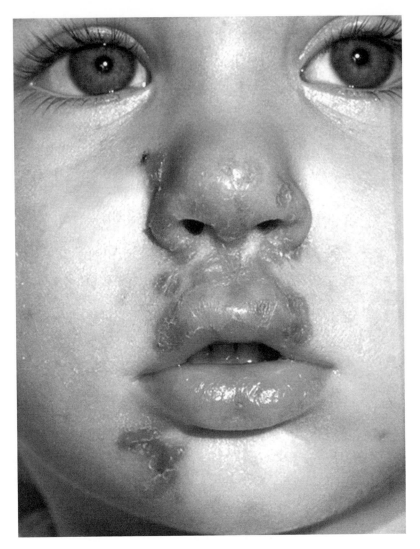

Figure 5-4 *Impetigo is commonly seen on the face.*
(T. Fitzpatrick, Color Atlas and Synopsis of Clinical Dermatology, 3e. Reproduced with permission of The McGraw-Hill Companies, 1996.)

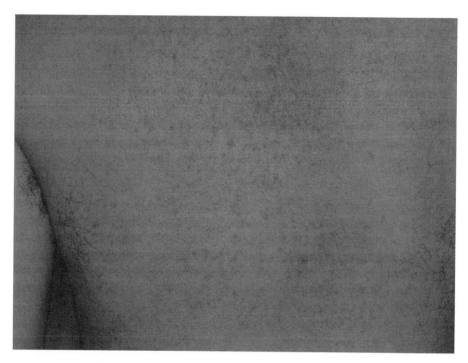

Figure 5-5 *Folliculitis on the back.*
(Courtesy Rube J. Pardo, M.D., Ph.D.)

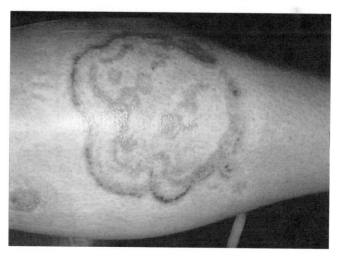

Figure 5-6 *Tinea corporis infection on the leg.*
(Courtesy Rube J. Pardo, M.D., Ph.D.)

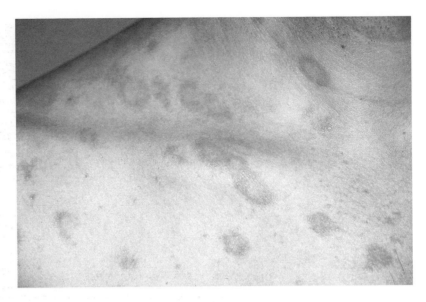

Figure 5-7 *Pityriasis rosea.*
(Courtesy Mark Lees Skin Care, Inc.)

Viral Infections

A virus is a parasite that cannot feed or reproduce on its own and requires a host cell to "live." **Viral infections** can be difficult to treat because the virus may hide from the host's immune system inside the host's own cells.

Viral warts occur when the virus enters the body through direct contact with the skin. Measles results from the virus gaining access through the respiratory system. Systemic infections like measles often affect a number of other body systems as well as the skin.

Venereal disease (VD) is a contagious disease acquired by contact with an infected person during sex. VD can be avoided by abstinence or practicing safe sex.

GLOVES

Keeping irritating substances away from the skin prevents allergies and related diseases. Wearing gloves is an excellent way to lower skin exposure. Excuses, such as "I need to feel the hair," "they're too uncomfortable," or "it's inconvenient," are common statements of justification.

There is no need to feel the hair while applying chemicals and no one can check the progress of a chemical application by feel. Feel the hair for texture and condition before the products are applied or after removal. Otherwise, always wear gloves.

GLOVES ARE THE SKIN'S BEST FRIEND

Rubber gloves are probably the last thing you'd suspect to cause allergic contact dermatitis. However, some hairstylists have become allergic to the chemicals found in rubber. Others develop sensitivities to the cornstarch used to make powdered gloves. Although these are not common occurrences, hairstylists should be aware of the possibility.

Sometimes the allergy is not from the glove but, instead, from moisture buildup between the glove and hand. When prolonged, skin wetness can create problems; using powdered gloves often eliminates the symptoms.

If you become sensitized to rubber gloves, there are other alternatives. Gloves can be obtained in a wide variety of materials. A dermatologist can advise which one is best suited to your condition.

Don't be fooled into believing you can't wear gloves because you're sensitive. Gloves will protect the skin and prevent chemicals from being absorbed into the bloodstream.

	Disposable Gloves
Material Type	**Benefits**
Vinyl	Inexpensive, exceptional sensitivity, and chemical resistance
Natural Latex	Inexpensive, improved strength, good sensitivity, and chemical resistance
Polyethylene	Lowest cost, but lower sensitivity, strength, and chemical resistance
Polyurethane	Excellent chemical resistance and strength, tough, sheer, and high sensitivity

Without question, wearing gloves can be uncomfortable and inconvenient. Painful rashes, blisters, open sores, and cracked, dry skin are even more uncomfortable. The long-term health risks of skin absorption can be inconvenient. Many hairstylists with extreme sensitivities to salon chemicals are forced to leave the profession. Wearing gloves is far less inconvenient than finding new employment. Besides, properly fitted gloves can be comfortable. Once you get in the habit of wearing gloves, you'll feel uncomfortable without them!

Today, hundreds of different types of gloves are available in dozens of materials. These range from gloves that reach the shoulders to individual finger gloves. You can choose powdered or powder-free, cotton-lined or unlined, straight or naturally curved fingers, and ultrasheer to heavy duty. Some gloves even have a rough texture for improved grip and handling ability.

Try different types of gloves to determine which is right for you. Companies that distribute safety equipment often provide assistance in choosing proper gloves (see Appendix for sources of safety information).

Thanks to new technology and increasing chemical awareness, there is no reason to risk your health. Skin disease is easily avoidable, but you must make an effort to protect yourself. Working safely is working smart!

REVIEW QUESTIONS

1. What is a common occupational disease for hairstylists?

2. Which is more dangerous to the skin, irritants or corrosives? Explain why.

3. Name the two most common types of skin diseases found on clients who patronize salons.

4. What is the difference between an irritant and an allergen (sensitizer)?

5. What irritant substance is most commonly used in the salon?

6. Which type of skin disease may take up to 48 hours to develop symptoms?

7. Define *sensitizer*.

8. At what stage in a cosmetology career are you at the greatest risk of developing irritant contact dermatitis? Why?

9. At what stage in a cosmetology career are you at the greatest risk of developing allergic contact dermatitis? Why?

DISCUSSION QUESTIONS

1. Carefully examine the list of different types of disposable gloves. Which glove do you feel offers the best combination of affordability, comfort, strength, and chemical resistance? Did you pick the same glove your classmates chose?

Chapter 6

The Growth and Structure of Hair

Key Terms

Amino acids
Arrector pili muscle
Cortex
Cuticle
Cysteine
Cystine
Dermal papilla
Disulfide bonds
End bonds
Follicle
Helix
Hydrogen bonds
Keratin
Medulla
Peptide bonds
Polypeptides
Proteins
Salt bonds
Side bonds
Stem cells

Learning Objectives

After completing this chapter, you should be able to:

- Understand how a hair follicle forms and grows.

- Describe the structure of hair.

- Describe hair's subfiber structure.

- Account for the physical properties of hair.

- Explain why keratin is cross-linked.

WHY DO WE NEED HAIR?

Our primitive ancestors depended on hair for warmth and protection, and although hair is no longer needed for survival, it still has an enormous impact on our psychology.

The social importance of hair is astounding. In the 1960s, hair length was not just a fashion statement but a political one as well. Some religions insist on complete removal of the hair, while others forbid cutting it. In some ancient civilizations, hair was a symbol of power, while in others it was considered a sign of wisdom.

According to the Bible, Samson's hair made him the strongest man on Earth, and cutting it was his downfall. In Japanese history, the importance of a woman's hair was second only to her life! A woman's immortal spirit was thought to be located in her hair. Even in modern times, the significance of hair and its styling is still deeply rooted in every culture.

The earliest records of hair growth studies come from the ancient Greeks. Aristotle noticed that eunuchs (men or boys deprived of the testes or external genitals) never lost their hair. Centuries later, Julius Caesar demanded that the Roman senate allow him to wear his laurel wreath at all times to hide his baldness. He also carefully groomed his hair to shield his bald spot from Cleopatra's view.

STRUCTURES OF THE SCALP

There are approximately 100,000 hair follicles in the scalp. Each of these follicles was created by a special relationship between the dermis and epidermis. As the scalp develops, certain changes take place. Look at Figure 6-1 and use your imagination to visualize the creation of a hair **follicle** (**FOL**-i-kel).

Follicle Formation

Before a hair follicle can develop, tissue cells must undergo a dramatic change (Fig. 6-2). First, a portion of the epidermis grows downward into dermal tissue creating a deep canal called the follicle. Deep in the dermis (just above the subcutaneous layer) this newly formed follicle canal wraps itself tightly around a small piece of dermis tissue. The epidermis almost completely surrounds this piece of dermis. This process of follicle formation happens about five million times on the average body.

Dermal Papilla

The small, cone-shaped piece of dermis tissue that bulges up into this new follicle canal is called the **dermal papilla** (pa-**PIL**-uh). Since the epidermal tissue that lines the follicle canal has no blood supply of its own, oxygen and nutrients are supplied by tiny capillaries located in the dermal papilla. Eventually, the epidermis tissue completely surrounds the papilla and forms a *hair bulb*. Capillaries remain attached to the bottom of the bulb. If you pull a hair from its follicle, you can see this bulb of dermis tissue (Figs. 6-3 through 6-7).

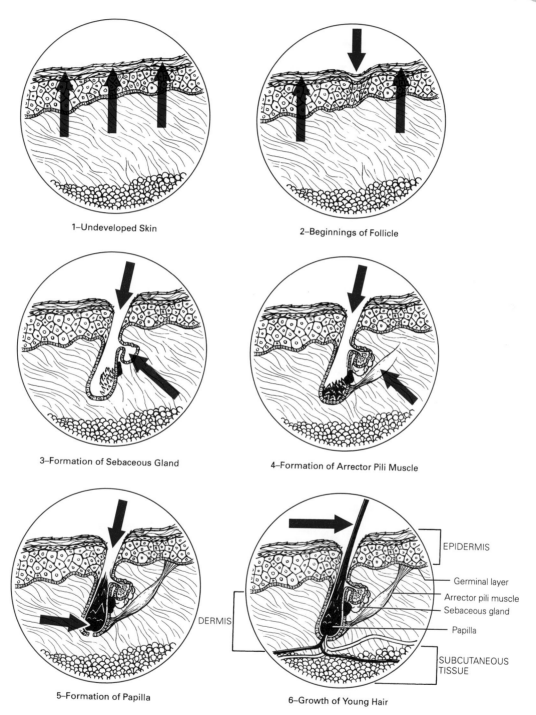

1–Undeveloped Skin

2–Beginnings of Follicle

3–Formation of Sebaceous Gland

4–Formation of Arrector Pili Muscle

5–Formation of Papilla

6–Growth of Young Hair

EPIDERMIS

Germinal layer

Arrector pili muscle

Sebaceous gland

Papilla

DERMIS

SUBCUTANEOUS TISSUE

Figure 6-1 *Origin of follicle and hair.*

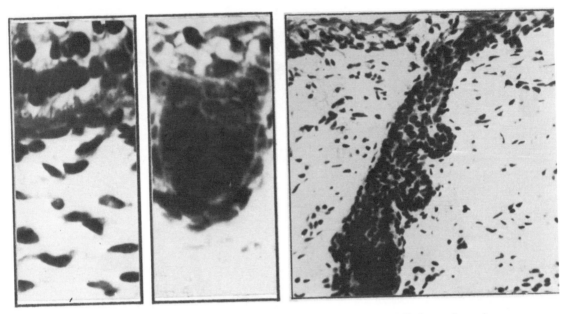

Figure 6-2 *Formation of follicle. Three stages in the development of hair follicles in the scalp approximately six months before birth.*
(Courtesy: Structure & Functions of Skin—*Academic Press*)

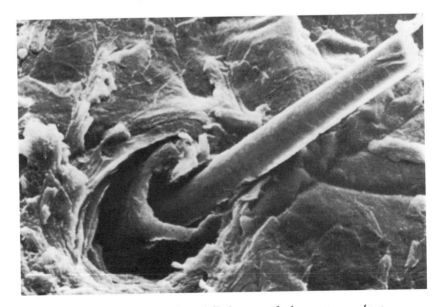

Figure 6-3 *Single hair growing from follicle, magnified 600 times. This is an excellent view of the follicle opening and the sheath around the base of the hair.*
(Courtesy: Gillette Company Research Institute, Rockville, Maryland)

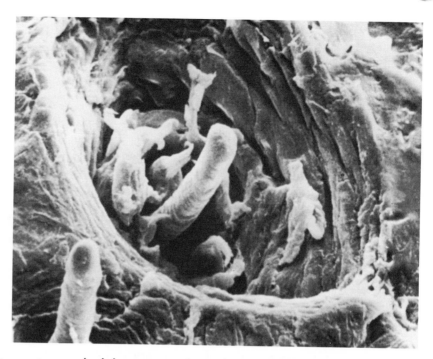

Figure 6-4 *Multiple hairs growing from what appears to be a single follicle, magnified 630 times. Notice follicle architecture, which is clearly shown in the center.*
(Courtesy: Gillette Company Research Institute, Rockville, Maryland)

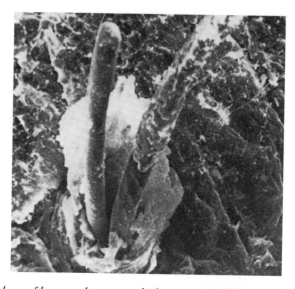

Figure 6-5 *Photo of human skin, magnified 360 times, showing two hairs emerging from what appears to be a single follicle. Also notice two fine hairs emerging from follicle in lower left corner.*
(Courtesy: Gillette Company Research Institute, Rockville, Maryland)

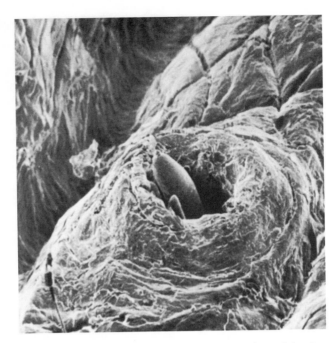

Figure 6-6 *Photo of two hairs just emerging from the surface of the skin, magnified 630 times. These represent two newly growing fibers.*
(Courtesy: Gillette Company Research Institute, Rockville, Maryland)

Hair Shaft

Hair grows from special types of cells called **stem cells.** Until late 1990, it was be-lieved that the stem cells were found in the epidermis cells surrounding the bulb and that the hair shaft grew upward from this "root." Scientific evidence now shows that this belief is incorrect.

Researchers at the University of Pennsylvania have found that stem cells come from a small bulge directly under the sebaceous (oil) glands. This bulge sits beside the follicle. This is where the hair shaft begins. These newly formed cells become quickly "keratinized." This means the cytoplasm of the cell is completely replaced by a special protein called **keratin.** As more and more keratinized cells are made, they are pushed into the follicle canal. After the entire canal becomes packed, a column of keratinized cells emerges from the follicle.

In chapter 4, we learned that newly formed epidermis cells in the skin are filled with cytoplasm and that each cell contains a nucleus. As a cell moves to-ward the skin's surface, the nucleus disappears and the cell becomes filled with ker-atin. The dead cells then flake off the skin's surface and are continually replaced by cells from below. A similar process occurs in the follicle. The keratinized cells

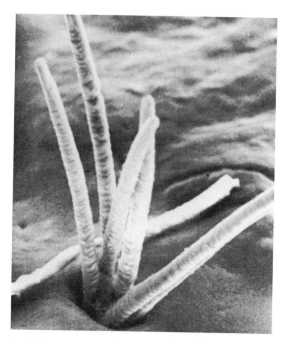

Figure 6-7 *Multiple hairs growing from what appears to be a single follicle, magnified 780 times, obtained from the forehead of a young male.*
(Courtesy: Gillette Company Research Institute, Rockville, Maryland)

of the hair shaft also contain no cytoplasm or nucleus. Hair cells die before the shaft of the hair ever pushes above the skin.

Other Special Structures

As the follicle canal is growing toward the dermis, other important changes are taking place. Several small, saclike bulges appear on the upper part of the follicle. One of the bulges becomes a sebaceous gland.

These glands make sebum. Sebum is secreted into the hair follicle and lubricates and conditions both the hair and skin. On the average, the body makes only one ounce of sebum every one hundred days. A little sebum goes a long way!

A second bulge on the follicle attaches to the **arrector pili muscle** (a-**REK**-tohr **PIGH**-ligh). This muscle can pull the hair shaft into an upright position. It also causes "goose bumps" or "goose flesh" on the skin. In primitive times, these muscles were important to survival. They could raise hair to an upright position allowing air to flow more freely across the skin to cool it and prevent over-heating. Goose bumps help control the flow of blood near the skin's surface and also cool the body (Fig. 6-8).

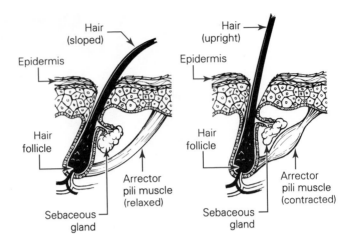

Figure 6-8 *Action of arrector pili muscle.*

STRUCTURE OF HAIR

From the outward appearance, hair is misleading. There is more to a strand of hair than meets the eye. Underneath the outer surface, there are many different layers. Each of these layers is important to healthy, beautiful hair. There are dozens of sub-layers: but only three separate and distinct main layers (Figs. 6-9 through 6-11).

1. Medulla

2. Cortex

3. Cuticle

Medulla

The **medulla** (me-**DUL**-uh) is the innermost portion of the hair shaft (Fig. 6-12). This section has between two and five rows of cells across. Usually, only thicker, coarse hair shafts contain a medulla.

All male beard hair contains a medulla. It is quite common for fine and naturally blond hair to lack a medulla. As far as cosmetology is concerned, the medulla is an "empty" air space and is not involved in any salon services.

Cortex

As much as 90 percent of the total weight of hair comes from the **cortex** (**KOR**-teks). The cortex gives the hair its strength, flexibility, elasticity, and color. The cortex is made of rectangular-shaped cells that are tightly bonded together. These cells are filled with keratin. The natural color of the hair is due to the pigment in

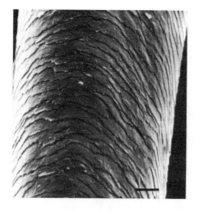

Figure 6-9 *Normal hair magnified 2,500 times.*
(Courtesy: Gillette Company Research Institute, Rockville, Maryland)

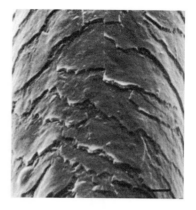

Figure 6-10 *Normal hair magnified 5,000 times.*
(Courtesy: Gillette Company Research Institute, Rockville, Maryland)

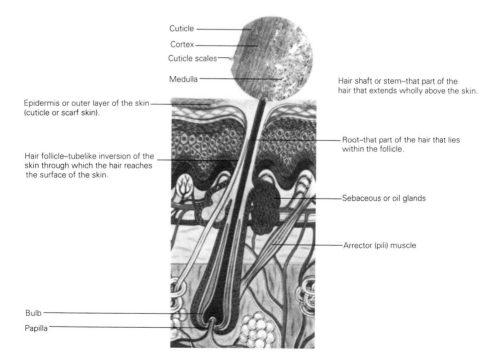

Cuticle
Cortex
Cuticle scales
Medulla

Hair shaft or stem–that part of the hair that extends wholly above the skin.

Epidermis or outer layer of the skin (cuticle or scarf skin).

Root–that part of the hair that lies within the follicle.

Hair follicle–tubelike inversion of the skin through which the hair reaches the surface of the skin.

Sebaceous or oil glands

Arrector (pili) muscle

Bulb
Papilla

Figure 6-11 *Cross section of skin and hair.*
(Courtesy: CEM and Gillette Company Research Institute, Rockville, Maryland)

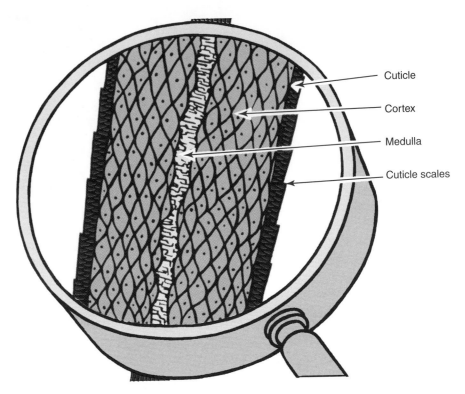

Figure 6-12 *Magnification of a cross section of hair.*

the cortex. For a natural-looking hair color it is necessary to get cosmetic coloring into this layer (Figs. 6-13 and 6-14).

Temporary and semi-permanent haircolor primarily coat the cuticle of the hair, which is transparent. Permanent haircolor can both lighten the natural color and deposit color within the cortex.

The elasticity of the hair is the result of the unique protein structure within the cortex. Wet setting, thermal styling, permanent waving, and chemical hair relaxing all take place within the cortex and would not be possible otherwise.

Cuticle

The cortex is surrounded by a single layer of overlapping transparent, scalelike cells of the **cuticle** (**KEW**-ti-kul). These scales overlap like shingles on a roof. A longitudinal section of hair shows that although the cuticle scales overlap, each individual cuticle scale is attached to the cortex (Fig. 6-15). This single layer of cuticle scales makes up the cuticle layer. Although when viewed on end, the scales can be seen to overlap, hair has only one overlapping, cuticle layer. A cross

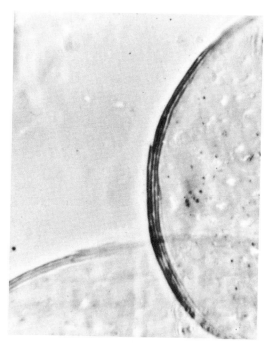

Figure 6-13 *Cross section of human hairs (magnified 500 times showing cortex with overlapping scales of cuticle).*
(Courtesy: Wool Industries Research Council)

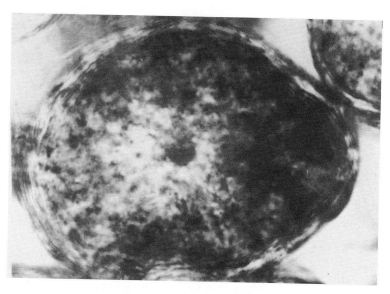

Figure 6-14 *Cross section of a straight hair. Note pigment in cortex and medulla (magnified 300 times).*
(Courtesy: Wool Industries Research Council)

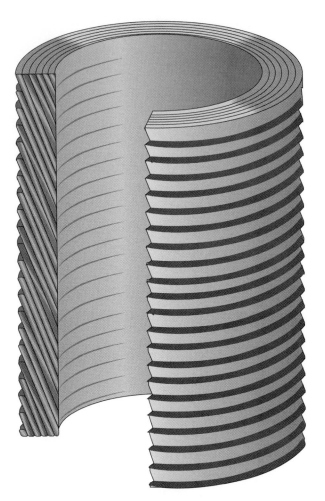

Figure 6-15 Cross section of hair showing that, although you can count six distinct layers of overlapping cuticle, each individual scale is attached to the cortex in one cuticle layer.

section of hair shows that when viewed on end, six distinct layers of overlapping cuticle scales can be seen (Fig. 6-15). The number of overlapping layers varies depending on the length of the cuticle scales. The hard cuticle protects the more delicate cortex and medulla. Without the cuticle layer, the cortex would become frayed and fall apart. The cuticle also acts as a barrier to chemicals such as tints and permanent wave lotions. This barrier is not impenetrable. Factors such as high pH and temperature can loosen the barrier. Since this layer is transparent, it is the pigment in the cortex which determines hair color (Figs. 6-16 through 6-19).

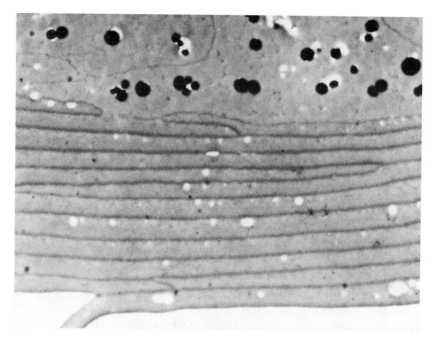

Figure 6-16 A photo of cuticle scales around the cortex, magnified 14,800 times. Eleven of cuticle scales layers can actually be counted overlaying the cortex. The dark black spots represent melanin granules in the fibers of the cortex.
(Courtesy: Gillette Company Research Institute, Rockville, Maryland)

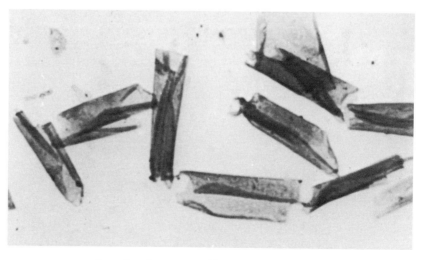

Figure 6-17 Cuticle scales after removal from hair shaft.
(Courtesy: Unilever Limited)

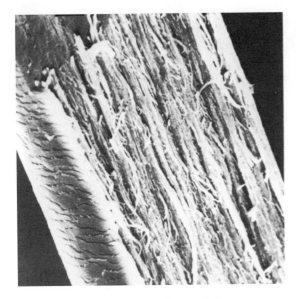

Figure 6-18 *Hair fiber with part of the cuticle stripped off exposing the cortex, magnified 1,470 times. Cortical fibrils can be clearly seen. Notice the vast difference in architecture of the interior of a fiber as compared to the surface.*
(Courtesy: Gillette Company Research Institute, Rockville, Maryland)

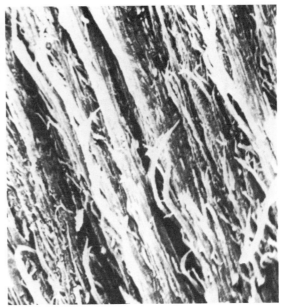

Figure 6-19 *This photo of the same hair structure in Fig. 6.18, magnified 4,200 times. This gives a closer view of the cortical fibers.*
(Courtesy: Gillette Company Research Institute, Rockville, Maryland)

SUBFIBERS AND PHYSICAL PROPERTIES OF HAIR

The combination of the medulla, cortex, and cuticle makes a fiber of hair, but it is the many subfibers which give the hair its physical properties.

Hair is a unique substance. Wet healthy hair can be stretched 40 to 50 percent and still return to its original length. Hair can withstand extreme temperatures and years of repeated stresses. The extraordinary properties of hair come from the complexities of its substructure. To understand these important properties fully, we must explore the basic foundation of each fiber.

The Protein Structure of Hair

Hair is approximately 91 percent **protein** (**PROH**-teen). Proteins are made of long chains of **amino acids** (uh-**MEE**-noh **AS**-udz) that are linked together end to end like pop beads. The chemical bond that links amino acids together is called a **peptide** (**PEP**-tyd) **bond** or **end bond**. A long chain of amino acids linked by peptide bonds is called a **polypeptide** (pahl-ee-**PEP**-tyd). Proteins are long, coiled, complex polypeptides made of amino acids. The shape of a coiled protein is called a **helix** (**HEE**-licks).

The Amino Acid Content of Hair

All the protein structures of hair are made from these eighteen amino acids.

Cysteic acid	Aspartic acid	Threonine
Arginine	Serine	Glutamic acid
Proline	Glycine	Alanine
Valine	Cystine	Methionine
Isoleucine	Leucine	Tyrosine
Phenylalanine	Lysine	Histidine

SIDE BONDS

The cortex is made of millions of polypeptide chains, which are cross-linked together by three types of **side bonds**: hydrogen bonds, salt bonds and disulfide bonds. These side bonds are essential to wet sets, thermal styling and permanent waving (Chapter 13, Permanent Waving).

A **hydrogen bond** is a special type of ionic bond. Within the structure of hair, a hydrogen bond occurs when a hydrogen atom, from the acid portion of an amino acid, is attracted to an oxygen atom, in the acid portion of another amino acid. Hydrogen bonds are easily broken by water or heat and are responsible for wet sets and thermal styling. Although individual hydrogen bonds are weak, there are so many of them is the hair that they account for about one third of the hair's total strength.

A **salt bond** is also an ionic bond. Within the structure of hair, a salt bond occurs when the negative charge of one amino acid is attracted to the positive charge of another amino acid. Salt bonds depend on pH and account for about one third of the hair's total strength. Salt bonds are easily broken by strong alkaline or acidic solutions.

A **disulfide** (dy-SUL-fyd) *bond* is a covalent bond, which is different from the ionic bonding of a hydrogen or salt bond. A disulfide bond joins the sulfur atoms of two neighboring cysteine amino acids to create cystine. Although there are fewer disulfide bonds than hydrogen or salt bonds, disulfide bonds are stronger and account for about one-third of the hair's total strength. Disulfide bonds are not broken by heat or water. Permanent waves and chemical hair relaxers work by creating chemical and physical changes in the hair's disulfide bonds.

Individual protein chains are cross-linked by side bonds to create tiny, invisible, threadlike fibers. At least nine of these fibers twist around each other to make larger bundles called *micro fibrils*. Dozens of micro fibrils, in turn, twist together to create larger *macro fibrils*. Finally, six macro fibrils intertwine to form *fibrils*, the cells of the cortex (Figs. 6-22 and 6-23).

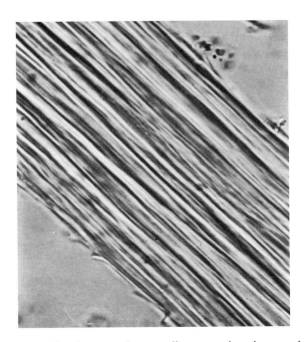

Figure 6-20 *Longitudinal section of cortex illustrating long keratin chain structure.*
(Courtesy: Wool Industries Research Council)

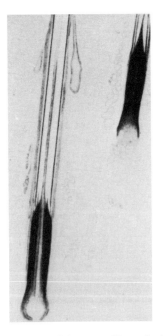

Figure 6-21 *Hair follicles showing soft keratin of hair (dark) and hard keratin (white).*
(Courtesy: Wool Industries Research Council)

KERATIN

Keratin is an important example of an insoluble, complex protein (Figs. 6–20 through 6–21). Hair is made almost entirely of this important substance. Keratin is made from eighteen different amino acids, including cystine and **cysteine** (**SIS**-ti-een) (uncross-linked cystine).

Cystine is the most abundant amino acid in hair. Cystine makes up nearly 18 percent of hair. With so many possibilities for making cross-linked disulfide (sulfur) bonds, cystine gives hair much of its strength. It is also responsible for causing hair to hold a permanent curl or relaxer.

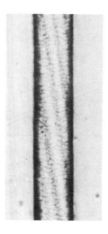

Figure 6-22 *Arrangement of twisted chains of hard keratin subfibers in hair cortex.*

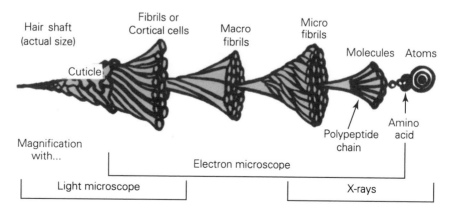

Figure 6-23 *Magnification of subfibers.*

This highly organized structure is designed much like the high-strength cables used to support suspension bridges. The polypeptide chains in keratin are both physically and chemically bound together. Millions of these keratinized cells are securely bonded together in the cortex and covered with a protective cuticle shield. This is how nature has created hair, a superstrength structure with amazing physical characteristics and chemical resistance!

REVIEW QUESTIONS

1. What type of cells line the walls of a hair follicle?

2. What are stem cells and why are they important?

3. Which of the three main layers of hair is most important to natural hair color? Why?

4. How do amino acids get to the dermal papilla?

5. Explain how, once amino acids reach the follicle, they become fibrils.

DISCUSSION QUESTIONS

1. Hairstylists and the hair styles they create have helped mold society and may influence future Americans for generations to come. How and why do you think this is possible?

2. Based on your understanding of the complex, subfiber structure of the cortex, does it seem reasonable that damaged hair can be "rebuilt" or "repaired" by using products that contain amino acids? (Hint: The answer is no; can you explain why?)

Chapter 7

The Properties of Hair

Key Terms

Anagen phase
Catagen phase
CHONS elements
Complimentary foods
Dihydrotestosterone
Essential amino acids
Eumelanin
Finasteride
Melanin
Melanocytes
Minoxidil
Nonessential amino acids
Phaeomelanin
Telogen phase
Terminal hairs
Vellus hairs

Learning Objectives

After completing this chapter, you should be able to:

- Understand the three phases of the hair growth cycle.

- Describe the different types of hair and where they are found.

- Explain normal daily hair loss.

- Describe the factors that influence hair color.

- Define hair density and its importance.

- Describe the chemical composition of hair.

- Understand the factors that influence hair growth.

GROWTH CYCLES

Like events in nature, hair growth also occurs in rhythms or cycles. Each complete cycle has three phases which are repeated again and again throughout life. The three cycles are called the **anagen phase,** the **catagen phase,** and the **telogen phase** (Fig. 7-1).

Anagen Phase

This is the growth part of the cycle. When hair is in the anagen phase, the stem cells actively manufacture new keratinized cells in the hair follicle. During this part of the cycle, hair cells are produced at staggering rates. It is believed that while in the anagen phase, hair cells are created faster than any other normal cell in the body. This part of the cycle generally lasts three to five years, but in extreme cases can last as long as ten years. Then it enters the next phase of the cycle.

Catagen Phase

This is the transition phase. During this phase, the follicle undergoes many striking changes. The follicle canal shrinks to about one-third of its length, leaving the dermal papilla far below. The lowermost part of the follicle is now located just below the sebaceous gland. The hair bulb disappears and the shrunken root end forms a rounded, brushlike *club.* The cells also stop making color pigments and the root takes on a milky white appearance. The dermal papilla shrinks and becomes a small compacted ball.

   Not all activity in this phase is destructive. During the catagen phase, the follicle is also preparing for new growth by making *germ cells.* Germ cells can be thought of as the "seeds" for new growth. The germ cells surround the club and await the signal to renew the anagen phase. The length of the catagen phase is only two to three weeks.

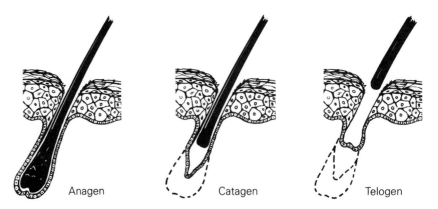

Anagen   Catagen   Telogen

Figure 7-1 *The anagen, catagen, and telogen phases of hair growth.*

Telogen Phase

Next, the follicle enters a resting stage called the telogen phase. Normally the old hair shaft is shed during this part of the cycle. Since the hair club may be anchored to the follicle walls, the hair may remain in place until the next anagen phase. Then it is pushed out by the new growth. The anagen phase lasts for about three to five years; consequently, the average lifetime of a hair shaft is four years.

The follicle will remain resting in the telogen phase for approximately three to six months. Then the entire cycle repeats itself on an average of once every four to five years.

HAIR TYPES

Two types of hair are found on the body: vellus and terminal. **Vellus hairs** (also called *lanugo hairs*) are short, fine, and silky soft. They almost never have a medulla or contain color pigments. On adults, they are usually found in places that are normally considered "hairless," i.e., forehead, eyelids, and bald scalp. The bodies of children and infants are covered with vellus hair, but it disappears after puberty. The vellus hair is replaced by thicker **terminal hair.** Women, however, retain 55 percent more vellus hairs than men.

Terminal (*tertiary*) **hair** is coarse and pigmented. It usually has a medulla and is easily distinguished from vellus hair.

The short, thick hairs that grow on the eyebrows and lashes are *primary terminal hairs*. After puberty, the fine vellus hairs are replaced by thicker, *secondary terminal hairs*. The same follicle is capable of producing both types of hair. Secondary terminal hair is mostly found on the scalp, beard, chest, back, legs, and pubic area. Frequently, when scalps begin to bald, the follicles stop making terminal hair and revert back to the vellus type (Fig. 7-2).

NORMAL HAIR LOSS AND GROWTH RATE

Normal Hair Loss

At any one time, 88 percent of scalp hair is in the anagen phase, one percent is in the catagen phase, and 11 percent is in the telogen phase. The scalp contains about 100,000 hairs on average, with slightly more for blonds and less for redheads. Although estimates of the rate of hair loss have long been quoted at 100 to 150 hairs per day, recent measurements indicate that the average rate of hair loss is closer to 35 to 40 hairs per day.

Growth Rate

In general, scalp hair grows faster on women than men. The average rate of growth is 0.36 mm/day (0.01417 inches/day) for women and 0.34 mm/day

GRADUAL LOSS OF HAIR

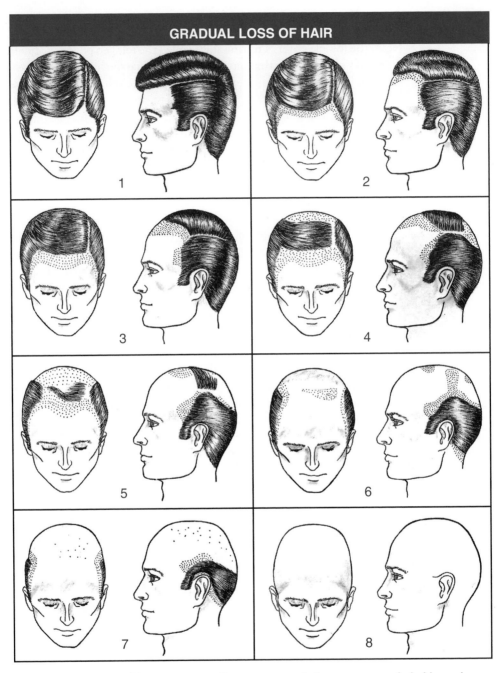

Figure 7-2 *Unless it is caused by some severe illness or unusual phenomenon, scalp baldness does not occur overnight. It is rather a gradual process, usually caused by some form of alopecia, during which the hair growth cycle is slowed down, interrupted, or discontinued entirely. This illustration shows the gradual loss of hair that occurs in the usual case of progressive baldness.*

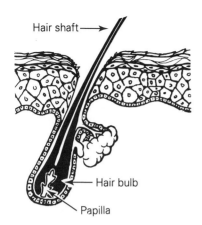

Figure 7-3 At an early stage of shedding, the hair shows its separation from the papilla.

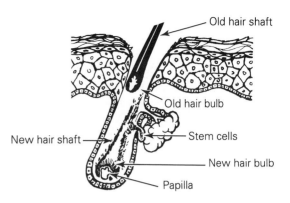

Figure 7-4 At a later stage of the hair shedding, a new hair is seen growing from the stem cells below the sebaceous gland.

(0.01339 inches/day) for men. Time-lapse photography shows that individual hairs grow at a constant rate day or night.

It has also been proven that shaving and cutting hair has absolutely *no ef-fect* on the rate of growth. Likewise, menstrual cycles have no effect on how rap-idly hair grows, but during pregnancy the growth rate slows slightly. Controlled studies show that scalp hair growth rates reach a maximum in the summer, while more hair shedding occurs in November.

If a follicle is pulled from the scalp, it takes about 130 days before a new hair emerges (Figs. 7-3 and 7-4).

The shedding of hair is not exactly regular; it is more noticeable in the morning and at certain other periods. No sensation of pain is felt when these hairs are pulled away from the scalp. The reason is that these hairs are not tightly bound and pull away easily. You may have noticed that when the scalp is brushed or combed a number of loose hairs are invariably found. These have detached them-selves from the scalp and may be seen on the brush, comb, coat, or pillow.

Each follicle has a definite age and when the hair reaches this natural limit, it falls out or is brushed or combed out. The follicle has a brief period of rest and then begins once more to produce a young new hair. On the scalp, this cycle of growth and replacement is from three to five years. The life span of the follicles of a woman's hair is about 25 percent longer than those of a man.

When the hair reaches its maximum age, an air space slowly develops be-tween the medulla and the top of the papilla. Following this, the cuticle of the hair is no longer formed by the outer cells of the papilla and the cortex shrinks in thickness. A short period later the complete hair bulb loosens and separates from the papilla. At this stage, the hair is known as a *bed-hair* and it lies loosely in the follicle. The papilla completely dies away and the follicle closes in over it. If the neck of the follicle is tight, it will continue to hold the bed-hair for a period of time.

The bed-hair may be pulled out by the daily brushing and combing, or it may be removed by shampooing or any other form of pulling or friction. Sometimes the bed-hair remains in the follicle until it is pushed out by the fresh, young hair.

Detached hair is known as *shed-hair*. Under the microscope the base of the shed-hair has a clublike, tattered appearance (Figs. 7-5 through 7-9).

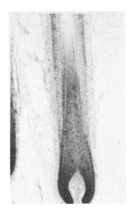 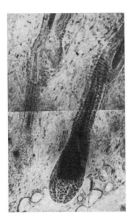 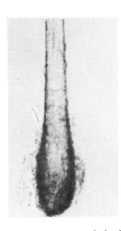

Figure 7-5 *A normal hair and follicle also showing hardening of cortex and cuticle (lighter areas).*

Figure 7-6 *A young follicle just starting to produce a hair. Note bed-hairs of previous cycles which have not been brushed or combed out.*

Figure 7-7 *A typical shed-hair illustrating club end.*

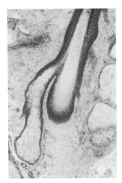 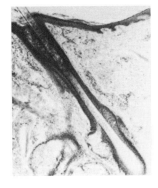

Figure 7-8 *A bed-hair in an old follicle. The follicle has shortened past it sebaceous gland.*

Figure 7-9 *An old hair in a dying follicle.*

Cutting a cross section of a hair reveals that it is not circular, but is instead irregular and *elliptical* (forming an oval). African-American black, curly hair is the most elliptical of all hair types. Asian hair is the closest to being round. The natural curl of hair is closely related to the cross-section shape. The more elliptical (flatter) the cross section, the curlier the hair (Figs. 7-10 through 7-14).

The strength of hair is remarkable. Each individual strand is actually stronger than an aluminum fiber of the same thickness! The average healthy head

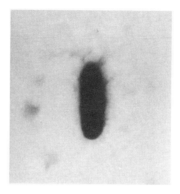

Figure 7-10 *Technology now provides microscopes that are so powerful that they can see inside a hair shaft. A single oval-shaped, blackish brown melanin molecule, such as the one shown, is the basis for all hair color.*
(Courtesy: Redken Laboratories, Inc.)

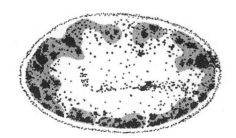

Figure 7-11 *A cross section of African-American black hair.*
(Courtesy: Redken Laboratories, Inc.)

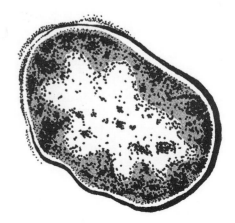

Figure 7-12 *A cross section of Caucasian hair.*
(Courtesy: Redken Laboratories, Inc.)

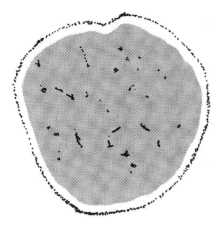

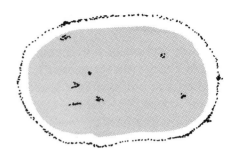

Figure 7-14 *A cross section of curly hair.*
(Courtesy: Redken Laboratories, Inc.)

Figure 7-13 *A cross section of straight hair.*
(Courtesy: Redken Laboratories, Inc.)

of hair, with 100,000 strands of hair, could lift over twelve tons. Because of its sub-fiber structure and disulfide bond cross-links, hair behaves much like reinforced wire cable.

Hair is also elastic and can be stretched, 40 to 50 percent of its length, without damage. However, hair should never be extended to more than 25 percent of its original length (Figs. 7-15 through 7-18).

Wetting the hair before stretching it greatly reduces the chance of damage. Compared to skin, hair is less resistant to water penetration. Normally, four percent to nine percent of a hair's weight is made up of water. However, the hair can absorb up to 40 percent of its normal dry weight in water. It will even absorb 30 percent of its weight directly from moisture in the air. When hair absorbs large amounts of moisture, it softens the hydrogen bonds and allows curls to relax.

Added water causes the hair to swell as much as 20 percent in diameter. Strong alkaline solutions (such as chemical relaxers) can increase the swelling to 100 percent. Chemicals that cause the hair to swell are often added to products to assist penetration of molecules that normally are too large to pass the cuticle.

Hair Body

Hair body is a combination of several hair characteristics. Many physical properties contribute to the hair body, including shaft diameter, texture, degree of curliness, density, moisture content, stiffness, and weight. Body is defined as the structural strength, volume, and resiliency of the hair.

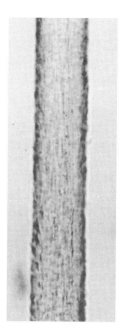

Figure 7-15 *Hair before stretching.*

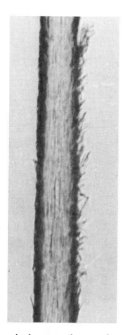

Figure 7-16 *Slight stretching is loosening cuticle scales.*

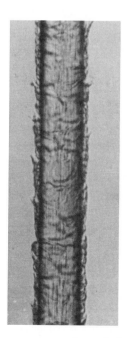

Figure 7-17 *Separation of cuticle from cortex has begun.*

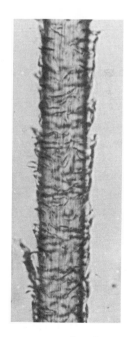

Figure 7-18 *Hair immediately prior to breakage; note the weakness due to excessive strain.*

Color

The pigment that gives natural color to hair and skin is called **melanin** (**MEL**-a-nin). The wide range of hair color is due to combinations of two types of melanin: **eumelanin** (yu-**MEL**-a-nin) and **phaeomelanin** (**FE**-o-mel-a-nin).

The type and amount of melanin in hair is an inherited, genetically controlled trait. Specialized cells called **melanocytes** (cytes = cells) produce all the melanin found in hair, skin, and eyes. Only completely white hair contains neither type of melanin. White is the actual color of keratin without the coloring influence of melanin.

Eumelanin is the most common type of melanin. This form gives hair shades from brown to black.

Phaeomelanin gives hair the yellowish-blond tones, ginger, and red colors.

Melanin pigments are found in the cortex. Both types of pigments are frequently present in the hair shaft. The ratio of eumelanin to phaeomelanin determines the hue seen in untreated hair. For example, red-blond tones such as copper-gold and medium chestnut brown result from mixtures of both pigments (Figs. 7-19 through 7-22).

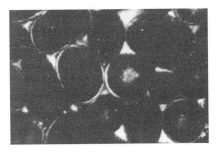

Figure 7-19 *Natural black straight hair (only black hairs). (These hairs absorb light intensely.)*

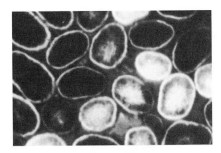

Figure 7-20 *Natural brown straight hair (contains black, brown, yellow hairs). (Note that there is no color in the cuticle.)*

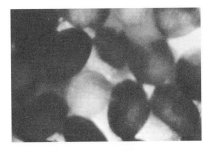

Figure 7-21 *Natural blond straight hair, golden shade (mostly dark hairs with lighter-colored hairs).*

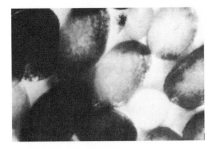

Figure 7-22 *Natural red straight coarse hair (auburn shade — contains yellow, red, brown, black hairs). (This hair has a large cortex with a thin cuticle layer.)*

Three factors determine all natural hair colors from light blond to jet black:

1. The thickness of the hair

2. The total number and size of pigment granules

3. The ratio of eumelanin to phaeomelanin

The number of pigment granules (*density*) is important. Not only does it affect the color of hair, but it can make changing the color easier or more difficult. The ebony black hair associated with African-Americans has the same type of melanin as Caucasian brown hair. The difference is that the melanin granules are twice as large in black hair. This gives a higher pigment density.

Blond hair has fewer and smaller phaeomelanin granules which are widely spread through the cortex. It would be easier to mask the effects of these pigments (low density) than to cover densely packed eumelanin granules. Bleaching hair actually destroys the melanin granules and removes their coloring influence (Fig. 7-23).

When the number of pigment granules begins to decrease naturally, graying becomes noticeable. This usually begins between 28 and 42 years old. Graying indicates the melanocytes are slowing down and making less melanin. Research shows that melanin production stops completely during the catagen and telogen phases (Fig. 7-24 and 7-25).

Normal hair color sometimes changes noticeably between 13 and 20 years old. This change is especially noticeable in blond, red, and light brown hair. These colors often begin to darken. This is due to increased melanin production. Higher pigment density causes darkening. Apparently, melanocytes vary the amount of pigment they produce according to age.

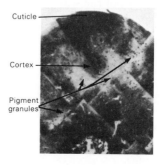

Cuticle

Cortex

Pigment
granules

Figure 7-23 *Pigment granules.*

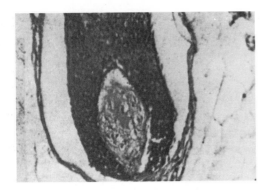

Figure 7-24 *Aging hair bulb with gray hair. Granules are formed but lack pigment.*
(Courtesy: Biology of Hair Growth—Academic Press)

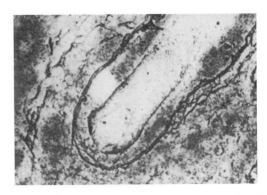

Figure 7-25 *Albino hair showing no granules of pigment in bulb.*
(Courtesy: Biology of Hair Growth—Academic Press)

Density

Hair density measures how many hairs are growing in a square inch of scalp. It tells how thick or full the hair is growing. Hair density varies widely among individuals, as well as races. The average hair density is about 2,200 hairs per square inch. Hair density is also influenced by cosmetic hair procedures, daily care, and disease/health.

- Hair density remains the same during pregnancy.
- Hair density is lower in women.
- Hair density decreases in both sexes after age fifty.
- Hair density is highest in young adults.
- Hair density decreases in chemically overprocessed hair.
- Hair density decreases with improper brushing techniques.

It is not practical to count hair on a client's head, but paying attention to the general, overall density can provide valuable information about the condition and health of the scalp. Blonds generally have the highest density and redheads have the lowest.

Diameter

Hair thickness is the diameter of each hair strand and can be classified as fine, medium, or coarse. Hair thickness is dependent on genetics and is known to vary based on racial background. Hair thickness not only varies from person to person, but also from strand to strand, on the same person's head.

It should be obvious that fine hair is fragile and the most susceptible to damage from salon services. As a general rule, fine hair will process faster and with less difficulty than medium or coarse hair.

Coarse hair is stronger than fine hair, for the same reason that a thick rope is stronger than a thin rope. Coarse hair has a larger diameter and will not only require more processing, but it may also be more resistant to that processing. It is usually more difficult for hair lighteners, haircolor, and permanent waving solutions to penetrate coarse hair (Figs 7-26 through 7-28).

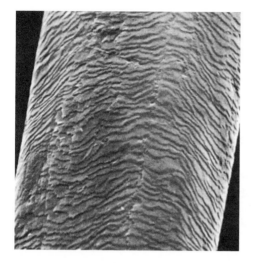

Figure 7-26 *Coarse hair magnified 1,200 times.*
(Courtesy: Gillette Company Research Institute, Rockville, Maryland)

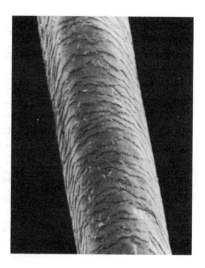

Figure 7-27 *Medium hair magnified 1,200 times.*
(Courtesy: Gillette Company Research Institute, Rockville, Maryland)

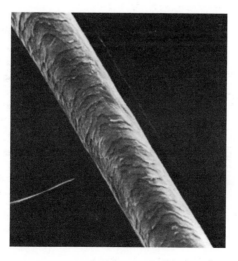

Figure 7-28 *Fine hair magnified 1,200 times.*
(Courtesy: Gillette Company Research Institute, Rockville, Maryland)

Chemical Composition

The protein in human hair is made of amino acids and those amino acids are made of elements. Human hair is composed of carbon, hydrogen, oxygen, nitrogen, and sulfur. These five elements are the major elements in skin and hair and are often referred to as the CHONS elements. Table 7-1 shows the relative ratios of each element in normal hair.

Factors That Influence Growth

Hair growth is not completely understood. For example, no one is sure what signal tells the follicle to leave the telogen phase and resume growth in the anagen phase. Still, several factors have been shown to influence hair growth on the scalp. Some of these are race, age, sex, season of the year, location on the body, nutrition, and hormones.

Pregnancy seems to disrupt the normal growth cycle of hair. Women usually have little hair loss during their pregnancy, but experience sudden and excessive shedding from three to nine months after delivery. Although this is can be traumatic to the new mother, the growth cycle quickly returns to normal.

Hair Loss Treatments

There are currently two drugs that have been proven to stimulate the growth of hair and are approved by the Food and Drug Administration (FDA).

1. **Topical Medication**

   Minoxidil is a topical medication that lowers blood pressure. This topical solution is applied to the scalp twice a day, and although it's greasy and inconvenient, it has been proven to stimulate hair growth. It's sold over the counter (OTC), as a non-prescription drug under the brand name *Rogaine*. Minoxidil is available for both men and women and comes in two different strengths: 2 percent regular and 5 percent extra strength. It is not known to have any adverse side effects. Although there are many advertisements to the contrary, there is no evidence that massage, physical stimulation, or any other topical treatment encourages hair growth.

TABLE 7-1	Average Elemental Composition of Hair[1]	
	Carbon	51%
	Hydrogen	6%
	Oxygen	21%
	Nitrogen	17%
	Sulfur	5% (from cystine)

2. Oral Medication

Hair growth is controlled by androgens that are converted to testosterone. Testosterone is converted to **dihydrotestosterone** (DHT) by the enzyme 5-alpha-reductase. At sexual maturity, DHT causes the vellus pubic hair in males and females to be converted to longer, thicker terminal hair. DHT also causes the facial hair of males to be converted to the longer, thicker, terminal hair we know as a beard.

Paradoxically, in male pattern baldness (androgenic hair loss) that occurs later in life, the same DHT causes the miniaturization of the terminal hair of the scalp to vellus hair. At the same time, DHT stimulates the vellus hair on the rest of the male body to become terminal hair. Men with male pattern baldness lose their scalp hair and grow thicker, longer, darker hair on the rest of the body, especially the upper arms and back.

Finasteride is an oral, prescription medication for men only. Finasteride is sold under the brand name *Propeca*. Finasteride inhibits the production of 5-alpha-reductase, the enzyme that reacts with (DHT) to cause male pattern baldness. Although Finasteride is more effective and convenient than Minoxidil, possible side effects include weight gain and loss of sexual function. These drugs are available for men only and only by prescription. Women may not use this treatment, and pregnant women or those who might become pregnant are cautioned not to touch the drug because of the strong potential for birth defects.

Amino Acids and Nutrition

Although more than 100 **amino acids** naturally occur, the proteins of all plants and animals are made from just 20 "common" amino acids. Eleven of the 20 common amino acids are called the **nonessential amino acids** because they can be synthesized by the body and don't have to be in our diet. The remaining nine are the **essential amino acids** that must be in our daily diet because they cannot be synthesized by the human body.

There is some confusion concerning histidine, which has long been considered an essential amino acid for infants but recently has also been shown to be essential for adults. Cystine and tyrosine may also be essential to some infants who may not be able to synthesize them due to liver damage.

11 NON-ESSENTIAL AMINO ACIDS

Alanine	Arginine	Asparagine
Aspartic acid	Glutamic Acid	Glutamine
Glycine	Serine	Proline
Cystine*	Tyrosine*	

*Cystine and tyrosine may be essential in some infants.

9 ESSENTIAL AMINO ACIDS	Histidine	Isoleucine	Leucine
	Lysine	Methionine	Phenylalanine
	Threonine	Tryptophan	Valine

Although meat, fish, poultry, eggs, and dairy products are complete proteins that provide all of the essential amino acids, they should be limited in the diet because they are also high in fat. Many plant sources are low in fat and also a good source of fiber, but they are not complete proteins because they all lack at least one of the essential amino acids. **Complimentary foods** are combinations of two incomplete proteins that provide all the essential amino acids and make a complete protein. Some complimentary proteins are peanut butter and bread, rice and beans, beans and corn, and black-eyed peas and cornbread.

If you eat an adequate amount of complete protein each day, there is no need to take amino acid or protein supplements. Remember that protein supplements in large amounts can be harmful, particularly to the kidneys (Fig. 7-29).

Other Nutritional Factors

It is tempting to believe that certain foods influence the growth of longer, stronger, or more beautiful hair. As nice as this sounds, there is no evidence that any specific food can improve hair or speed its growth. Unfortunately, what you eat (or don't eat) can have many negative effects.

Both skin and hair require vitamins for healthy development, but vitamin supplements can do more harm than good! Excessive amounts of Vitamin A, for instance, appear to cause hair loss and can be toxic.[2]

The solution is proper nutrition. Eating correctly is the most important thing you can do to keep healthy. Vitamin supplements are not necessary if you eat properly. Vitamins don't correct problems that are caused by improper eating habits.

No vitamin supplement can substitute for eating wisely. In fact, vitamins can harm you if taken excessively. If you suspect you need a dietary supplement, get advice from a qualified medical doctor.

Eat a wide range of foods in moderation, from each of the basic food groups.

1. C. Zviak, *The Science of Hair Care* (New York: Marcel Dekker, Inc., 1986).
2. Masusle, R. and Zaun, H., *Fortschr. Med.*, 1972, 90:687.

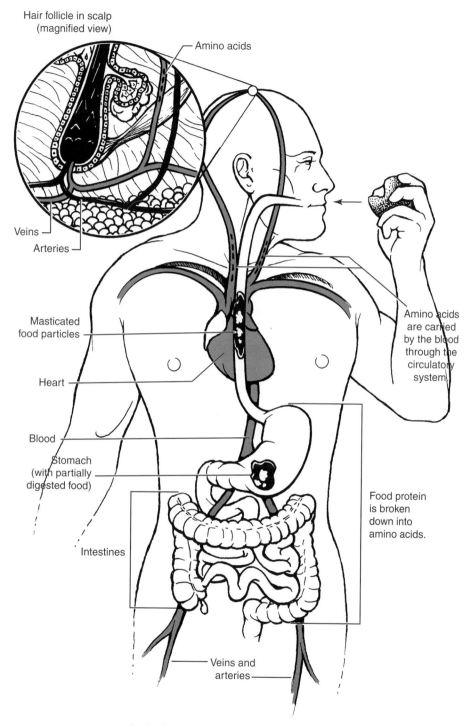

Hair follicle in scalp
(magnified view)

Amino acids

Veins

Arteries

Masticated
food particles

Heart

Blood

Stomach
(with partially
digested food)

Intestines

Veins and
arteries

Amino acids
are carried
by the blood
through the
circulatory
system.

Food protein
is broken
down into
amino acids.

Figure 7-29 *Digestion converts the food we eat into a form that can supply nourishment to the skin and hair.*

REVIEW QUESTIONS

1. What are the three phases of hair growth, and how long does each phase last?

2. Which grows faster, men's hair or women's?

3. On the average, how long will most hairs remain in the scalp?

4. Which type of hair is found on the head and legs of both sexes?

5. Using the information found in this chapter, estimate how long the average hair would grow on a woman in one year. Then do the same for an average male. How do they compare?

6. What combination of pigments causes light chestnut brown hair?

7. What effect do chemical relaxer applications have on hair diameter?

8. Why would light blond hair be easier to color than dark blond hair?

9. If a client's scalp contains 100,000 hairs, use the average density of hair (given in this chapter) to figure out how many square inches are in the entire scalp.

DISCUSSION QUESTIONS

1. Hair comes in a variety of diameters. What factors (there are several) do you think influence the diameter of the hair? For example, could a hair shaft be wider than its follicle canal?

2. What do you suppose would happen if the length of a client's anagen phase was cut in half and his or her telogen phase lasted for one year?

3. If shaving or cutting hair has no effect on the rate of hair growth, why does hair seem to grow so fast after a shave, but so slowly when a man is growing a beard?

Chapter 8

General Chemistry

Key Terms

Atoms
Chemical change
Chemical compounds
Chemistry
Compound molecules
Organic chemistry
Elemental molecules
Elements
Emulsions
Immiscible
Inorganic chemistry
Matter
Miscible
Mixtures
Molecules
Physical change
Pure substance
Solute
Solutions
Solvent
Suspensions
States of matter

Learning Objectives

After completing this chapter, you should be able to:

- Describe the classification and structure of matter.

- Understand the difference among solutions, suspensions, and emulsions.

- Explain how a physical change differs from a chemical change.

- List the properties of matter.

INTRODUCTION

Scientists refer to chemistry as the "Central Science" because it is essential to the study of all other sciences. Although you may not think so, chemistry is just as essential to hairstyling. None of the services performed in today's salon would be possible without chemistry.

Wet sets, thermal styling, permanent waving, and chemical hair relaxing rely on breaking and reforming the hair's side bonds with heat and chemicals (Chapter 13, Permanent Waving). All haircoloring services rely on chemicals. Chemical reactions develop the dye in oxidation haircolors and make it possible to lighten natural hair color (Chapter 12, Haircoloring). Maintaining healthy hair, skin, and scalp wouldn't be possible without the chemistry of shampoos and conditioners and there would be far fewer styling options without some type of setting lotion or hairspray (Chapter 10, Shampoos, Conditioners, and Styling Aids).

CHEMISTRY

Chemistry is the science of the structure and properties of matter and the changes it undergoes. There are two main branches of chemistry: organic chemistry and inorganic chemistry.

Organic Chemistry

Organic chemistry is the study of substances that contain the element carbon. All things that are, or ever were, alive contain carbon. You have probably heard the term organic incorrectly used to imply natural. That is a common mistake because of the association between the term organic and living, but organic does not mean natural. The term organic only means that the substance contains the element carbon. Most organic substances will burn. Plants, animals, gasoline, motor oil and plastics are all organic substances.

Inorganic Chemistry

Inorganic chemistry is the study of substances that do not contain carbon. Inorganic substances are not, and never were, alive. Inorganic substances will not burn. Metals, minerals, and ammonia are inorganic substances. The water we drink and the air we breathe are also inorganic. Inorganic does not mean unnatural or unhealthy.

MATTER

Matter is anything that has volume (occupies space) and mass (weight). Anything that you can see, touch, taste, and smell is matter. Although we can see visible light, color, and electric sparks, they are all forms of energy. Energy is not matter because it doesn't occupy space or have mass.

Elements

Elements are substances that cannot be separated into simpler substances by chemical means. There are 109 different elements known today and each has its own distinctive physical and chemical properties (Figs. 8-1 and 8-2). About 90 of the 109 elements occur naturally. The remaining elements have only been produced by artificial means. All the matter in the universe is made from these one hundred and nine different elements.

Atoms

Atoms are the basic building blocks of all matter. All matter is composed of atoms. An atom is the smallest particle of an element that retains the properties of that element. Atoms are the smallest units of matter and cannot be divided into simpler substances by chemical means. The word atom is derived from the Greek word *atomos*, which means indivisible.

Atoms are the structural units of the elements that makeup matter. The atoms of each element are different in structure from the atoms of all other elements. The structural differences of the 109 different atoms account for the 109 different elements and their properties.

Atoms can be compared to the letters of the alphabet (e.g., A, B, C, D). Each of the 26 letters in the English alphabet has a different structure that makes

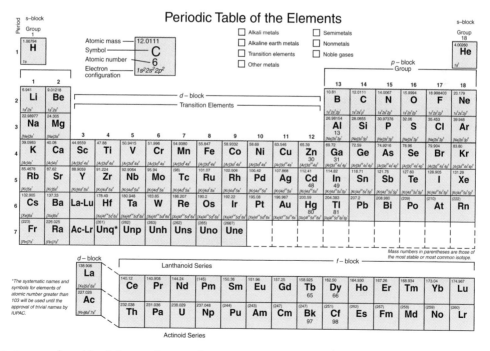

Figure 8-1 *Periodic table of the 109 known elements.*

Element	Symbol	Number	Element	Symbol	Number
Hydrogen	H	1	Barium	Ba	56
Helium	He	2	Lanthanum	La	57
Lithium	Li	3	Cerium	Ce	58
Beryllium	Be	4	Praseodymium	Pr	59
Boron	B	5	Neodymium	Nd	60
Carbon	C	6	Promethium	Pm	61
Nitrogen	N	7	Samarium	Sm	62
Oxygen	O	8	Europium	Eu	63
Fluoride	F	9	Gadolinium	Gd	64
Neon	Ne	10	Terbium	Tb	65
Sodium	Na	11	Dysprosium	Dy	66
Magnesium	Mg	12	Holmium	Ho	67
Aluminum	Al	13	Erbium	Er	68
Silicon	Si	14	Thulium	Tm	69
Phosphorus	P	15	Ytterbium	Yb	70
Sulfur	S	16	Lutetium	Lu	71
Chlorine	Cl	17	Hafnium	Hf	72
Argon	Ar	18	Tantalum	Ta	73
Potassium	K	19	Tungsten	W	74
Calcium	Ca	20	Thenium	Re	75
Scandium	Sc	21	Osmium	Os	76
Titanium	Ti	22	Iridium	Ir	77
Vanadium	V	23	Platinum	Pt	78
Chromium	Cr	24	Gold	Au	79
Manganese	Mn	25	Mercury	Hg	80
Iron	Fe	26	Thallium	Tl	81
Cabalt	Co	27	Lead	Pb	82
Nickel	Ni	28	Bismuth	Bi	83
Copper	Cu	29	Polonium	Po	84
Zinc	Zn	30	Astatine	At	85
Gallium	Ga	31	Radon	Rn	86
Germanium	Ge	32	Francium	Fr	87
Arsenic	As	33	Radium	Ra	88
Selenium	Se	34	Actinium	Ac	89
Bromine	Br	35	Thorium	Th	90
Krypton	Kr	36	Protactinium	Pa	91
Rubidium	Rb	37	Uranium	U	92
Strontium	Sr	38	Neptunium	Np	93
Yttrium	Y	39	Plutonium	Pu	94
Zirconium	Zr	40	Americium	Am	95
Niobium	Nb	41	Curium	Cm	96
Molybdenum	Mo	42	Berkelium	Bk	97
Technetium	Tc	43	Californium	Cf	98
Ruthenium	Ru	44	Eisteinium	Es	99
Rhodium	Rh	45	Fermium	Fm	100
Palladium	Pd	46	Mendelevium	Md	101
Silver	Ag	47	Nobelium	No	102
Cadmium	Cd	48	Lawrencium	Lr	103
Indium	In	49	Rutherfordium	Db	104
Tin	Sn	50	Dubnium	Db	105
Anitomy	Sb	51	Seaborgium	Sg	106
Tellurium	Te	52	Bohrium	Bh	107
Iodine	I	53	Hassium	Hn	108
Xenon	Xe	54	Meitnerium	Mt	109
Cesium	Cs	55			

Figure 8-2 List of elements by atomic number.

that letter different and identifies it. All the words in the English language are a combination of two or more of those 26 letters. All of the great works of American literature were written using only 26 different letters.

MOLECULES

Just as words are made by combining letters, molecules are made by combining atoms. **Molecules** are combinations of two or more atoms that are joined together chemically. The two types of molecules are: elemental molecules and compound molecules.

Elemental Molecules

Elemental molecules are chemical combinations of two or more atoms of the same element. When all the atoms that form a molecule are the same, the molecule is still an element and it is called an elemental molecule. The oxygen in the air that we breathe is the elemental molecule O_2, and the ozone in the atmosphere, that protects us from ultraviolet radiation, is the elemental molecule O_3. If molecules were like words in the English language, elemental molecules would look like this: AA, BBB, or CCCC.

Compound Molecules

Compound molecules are chemical combinations of two or more atoms of different elements. When two or more of the atoms that make a molecule are different, the molecule is a compound and called a compound molecule. Sodium chloride (NaCl), or common table salt, is a compound molecule that is a chemical combination of one atom of sodium (Na) and one atom of chlorine (Cl). If molecules were like words in the English language, compound molecules would look like this: AB, BAB, or CACC.

THE STATES OF MATTER

All matter exists in one of three different forms: solid, liquid, or gas. These three different physical forms are called the **states of matter**. The form in which matter appears is dependent on temperature.

Like most other substances, water (H_2O) can exist in all three states of matter, depending on its temperature. Ice turns to water as it melts and water turns to steam as it boils. The form of the water is different because of a change of state, but it is still water (H_2O). It is not a different chemical. It is the same chemical in a different form (Figs. 8-3 and 8-4).

Solids have a definite volume (size) and a definite shape. Ice is an example of a solid. Ice has a definite size and shape. Ice is solid water (H_2O) at a temperature of less than 32°F/0°C.

Liquids have a definite volume but not a definite shape. Water is an example of a liquid. Water has a definite size but does not have a definite shape. Water is liquid water (H_2O) at a temperature above 32°F/0°C and below 212°F/100°C.

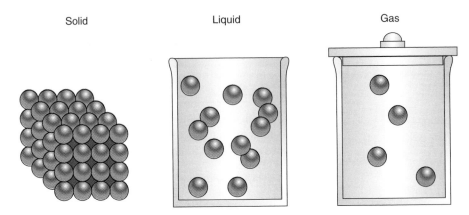

Solid   Liquid   Gas

Figure 8-3 *The three states of matter, solid, liquid and gas.*
(Reprinted with permission of PADI Americas)

Gases don't have a definite volume or a definite shape. Steam is an example of a gas. Steam doesn't have a definite size or a definite shape. Steam is gaseous water (H_2O) at a temperature at or above 212°F/100°C.

PHYSICAL AND CHEMICAL PROPERTIES

Every substance has a unique set of properties that allow us to identify it. These properties of matter can be grouped into physical properties and chemical properties.

Physical Properties

Physical properties are those characteristics that can be determined without a chemical reaction and without a chemical change in the identity of the substance. Physical properties include color, odor, weight, density, melting point, boiling point, and hardness. The color and weight of an object can be observed without a chemical reaction or a chemical change in the identity of the substance.

Chemical Properties

Chemical properties are those characteristics that can only be determined with a chemical reaction and will cause a chemical change in the identity of the substance. Chemical properties include the ability of iron to rust and wood to burn. In both of these examples, oxidation is the chemical reaction that creates a chemical change in the identity of the substance. The iron is chemically changed to

Types	Examples	Definition	Use in Cosmetology
PHYSICAL	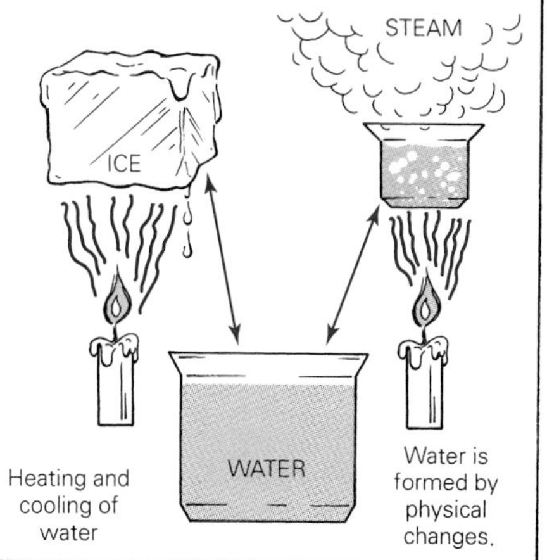 ICE STEAM Heating and cooling of water WATER Water is formed by physical changes.	Changes of a substance in form from solid-liquid-gas state. No new substance is formed. Action is easily reversible. Rate of change is simply controlled.	Setting, finger waving, etc. Hair is softened by setting agents – then hardened into waves by drying.
CHEMICAL	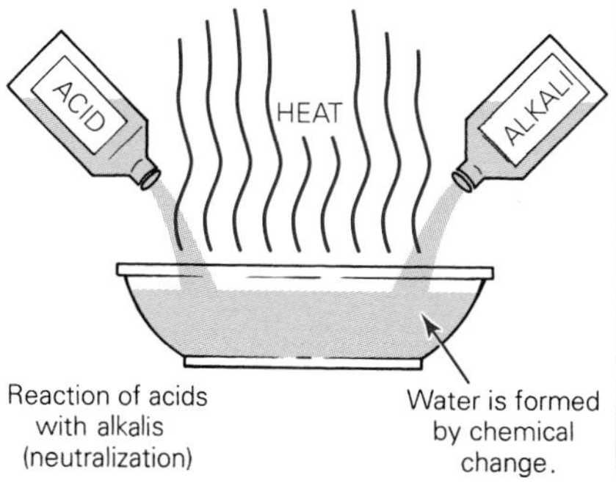 ACID HEAT ALKALI Reaction of acids with alkalis (neutralization) Water is formed by chemical change.	Permanent changes with formation of new substances. Action is NOT easily reversible. Rate of change must be controlled by: a. Temperature b. Concentration c. Time d. pH of solution in contact with the hair	COLD WAVING Keratin in cortex is chemically changed by waving solutions. Waves made permanent by reaction of neutralizers on changed keratin. BLEACHING Bleaches react with hair pigments to reduce color. TINTING Reaction of developer with tint bases forms tint pigments.

Figure 8-4 *Physical and chemical changes. Acid-alkali neutralization.*

rust and the wood is chemically changed to charcoal. The rust and charcoal are the products of the chemical reaction. They are different chemicals with different properties.

PHYSICAL AND CHEMICAL CHANGES

Matter can be changed in two ways. Physical forces create physical changes and chemical reactions create chemical changes (Fig. 8-4).

Physical Change

A **physical change** is a change in the form, or the physical properties, of a substance. A physical change is the result of physical forces. A physical change does not involve a chemical reaction and no new chemicals are formed. A change of state is an example of a physical change. Solid ice undergoes a physical change when it melts to liquid water. This is a physical change because ice and water are the same chemical (H_2O). There is no chemical reaction and no new chemicals are formed.

Temporary haircolor is an example of a physical change. Temporary haircolor changes the appearance of the hair by physically adding color molecules to the surface of the hair. Although the hair appears to be a different color, there is no change in the chemical structure of the hair. There is no chemical reaction and no new chemicals are formed.

Chemical Change

A **chemical change** is a change in the chemical properties of a substance. A chemical change is the result of a chemical reaction. The products created by a chemical reaction are new chemicals. Oxidation is an example of a chemical reaction that causes a chemical change. Iron undergoes a chemical reaction and a chemical change when it rusts. The iron changes chemically, combining with oxygen from the air, to produce a new substance called rust. This is a chemical change because iron and rust are not the same chemical. This is a chemical reaction and a new chemical is formed.

Permanent hair color is an example of a chemical change. Permanent haircolor changes the chemical structure of the color by chemically developing the dye and chemically adding color to the internal structure of the hair. The hair is a different color because of changes in the chemical structure of both the dye and the hair. This is a chemical reaction and new chemicals are formed.

PURE SUBSTANCES, COMPOUNDS, AND MIXTURES

All matter can be classified into one of two categories: either a pure chemical substance or a physical mixture (Figs. 8-5 and 8-6).

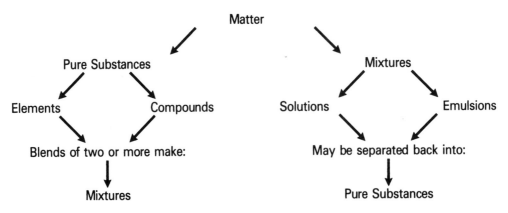

Figure 8-5 *Classification of Matter.*

Pure Substances

A **pure substance** is matter that has a fixed chemical composition, definite proportions, and distinct properties. Elements and chemical compounds are the two types of pure substances. Elemental molecules contain two or more atoms of the same element that are united chemically. Elemental molecules are pure substances. Aluminum foil is an example of a pure substance. Aluminum foil is composed only of atoms of the element aluminum. The properties of aluminum foil are the properties of the element aluminum.

Chemical Compounds

Chemical Compounds are combinations of two or more elements united chemically with a fixed chemical composition, definite proportions, and distinct properties. Chemical compounds are the result of a chemical reaction. The elements that are united in chemical compounds give up their own chemical identity and properties. The properties of chemical compounds are much different than the properties of the elements from which they were made.

Water (H_2O) is a chemical compound. A water molecule is composed of two atoms of the element hydrogen (H) and one atom of the element oxygen (O). These proportions are definite and any other combination is not water. When these two gases are joined together chemically they make the liquid, water. Water is a chemical compound with different properties than the elements oxygen and hydrogen from which it is made. Just like water, all chemical compounds are pure substances.

Mixtures

Mixtures are combinations of two or more substances united physically, without a fixed composition and in any proportions. Mixtures are not the result of a chemical

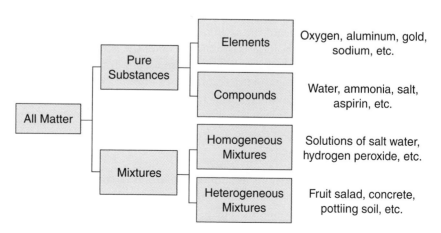

Figure 8-6 *Pure substances and mixtures.*

reaction. In a physical mixture, each substance retains its own identity and its own distinct properties. The properties of mixtures are a combination of the substances from which they are made. Pure air is a mixture of gases, mostly nitrogen and oxygen.

Fruit salad is a physical mixture of different types of fruits. Fruit salad can be made from many different types of fruits, mixed in any proportions. Fruit salad is a physical mixture. A chemical reaction is not involved and no new chemicals are formed. The properties of the fruit salad are the combined properties of the fruits in the mixture. The properties of the individual fruits are not changed; they are just mixed together. Although collectively it's fruit salad, we can still identify each individual type of fruit and physically separate each one (Figs. 8-5 and 8-6).

SOLUTIONS, SUSPENSIONS, AND EMULSIONS

Solutions, suspensions, and emulsions are all mixtures of two or more different substances. The distinction between solutions, suspensions, and emulsions is dependent on the size of the particles and the solubility of the components.

Solutions

Solutions (soh-**LOO**-shuns) are uniform mixtures of two or more mixable substances. A **solute** (**SOL**-yoot) is any substance that is dissolved into a solvent to form a solution. A **solvent** (**SOL**-vent) is any substance that dissolves the solute to form a solution. If a gas or a solid is dissolved in a liquid, the gas or solid is the solute and the liquid is the solvent. When one liquid is dissolved in another liquid, the minor component is usually the solute and the major component is the solvent.

Miscible (**MIS**-eh-bel) liquids are mutually soluble. Water and alcohol are examples of miscible (mixable) liquids. **Immiscible** liquids are not mutually soluble. Water and oil are examples of immiscible (nonmixable) liquids. You've probably heard the saying, "oil and water don't mix."

Solutions contain particles the size of a small molecule that are invisible to the naked eye. Solutions are usually transparent although they may be colored. Solutions do not separate on standing. Salt water is a solution of a solid dissolved in a liquid. Water is the solvent that dissolves the salt and holds it in solution. Air, salt water, and hydrogen peroxide are examples of solutions.

Suspensions

Suspensions are uniform mixtures of two or more substances. Suspensions differ from solutions due to the size of the particles. Suspensions contain larger particles than solutions. The particles in a suspension are large enough to be visible to the naked eye. Suspensions are not usually transparent and may be colored. Suspensions have a tendency to separate over time.

Oil and vinegar salad dressing is an example of a suspension with oil suspended in vinegar. Salad dressing will separate on standing and should be shaken well before use. Many of the lotions used by hairstylists are suspensions and should be shaken or mixed well before use. Salad dressing, paint, and aerosol hair spray are examples of suspensions.

Emulsions

Emulsions (ee-**MUL**-shuns) are suspensions (mixtures) of two immiscible liquids held together by an emulsifying agent. The term emulsify means "to form an emulsion," which is a suspension of one liquid dispersed in another. Although emulsions have a tendency to separate over time, a properly formulated emulsion, that is stored correctly, should be stable for at least three years. Without adequate dispersion, emulsions can become unstable and break (separate) into two insoluble layers.

Mayonnaise is an oil-in-water emulsion of two immiscible liquids. Although oil and water are immiscible, the egg yolk in mayonnaise emulsifies the oil droplets and disperses them uniformly in the water. Without the egg yolk as an emulsifying agent, the oil and water would separate into two insoluble layers. Mayonnaise should not separate on standing. Many of the lotions and creams used by hairstylists are emulsions. Mayonnaise, cold cream, shampoos, and conditioners are examples of emulsions. Emulsions will be covered in more detail in Chapter 10, Shampoos, Conditioners, and Styling Aids.

REVIEW QUESTIONS

1. Define the word chemical.
2. List the three states of matter.
3. What is the difference between an emulsion and a suspension?
4. How do compounds differ from elements? How do atoms differ from molecules?

DISCUSSION QUESTIONS

1. Make a list of organic substances that are poisonous.
2. Make a list of inorganic substances that are healthy.
3. An increase in temperature causes ice to melt. What is heat? Why does adding heat make ice melt?

Chapter 9

Advanced Chemistry

Key Terms

Acids
Alkalis
Anions
Cations
Hydrogen ion
Hydroxide ion
Ions
Logarithm
Oxidation
pH scale
Reduction

Learning Objectives

After completing this chapter, you should be able to:

- Understand acids, alkalis, and pH.

- Describe how pH influences the skin, scalp, and hair.

- Explain oxidation and reduction reactions.

- Describe how to safely handle corrosives and oxidizers.

INTRODUCTION

This chapter builds upon the concepts presented in Chapter 8, General Chemistry. The concepts of pH and oxidation-reduction are essential to haircoloring, permanent waving and chemical hair relaxers.

WATER AND pH

You may already know that the pH scale ranges from 0 to 14. A pH of 7 indicates a neutral solution, a pH below 7 indicates an acidic solution, and a pH above 7 indicates an alkaline solution. Although this says something about how pH is measured, it doesn't say anything about what pH is. You may also know that acids contract and harden the hair and alkalis soften and swell the hair. Although this says something about how the hair reacts to acids and alkalis, it still doesn't say anything about what pH really is.

We can't study pH without first learning a little about ions. An **ion** (**EYE**-on) is an atom or molecule with an electrical charge. When a molecule ionizes, it splits in two, creating a pair of ions with opposite electrical charges. An ion with a negative electrical charge is an **anion** (**AN**-eye-on). An ion with a positive electrical charge is a **cation** (**KAT**-eye-on). The pH scale measures ions.

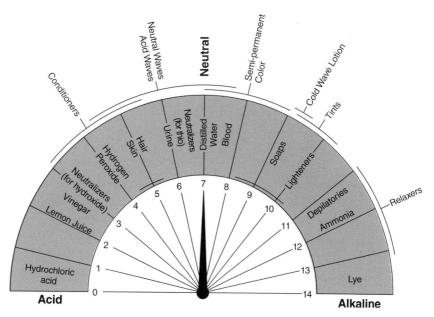

Figure 9-1 *Average pH values.*

Why is the pH of pure water neutral and what does that mean? A water molecule (H_2O) is composed of two hydrogen atoms and one oxygen atom. But some of the water molecules don't stay together as water molecules (H_2O). Because of the natural ionization of water, some of the water molecules (H_2O) ionize (split) into two separate ions: H^+ and OH. (See Fig. 9-2.)

A water molecule can be expressed as H_2O and the natural ionization of water can be expressed as:

$$H_2O \rightarrow H^+ + OH^-$$

That same water molecule can also be expressed as HOH, and the auto-ionization of water can be expressed as:

$$HOH \rightarrow H^+ + OH^-$$

The H^+ ion is the **hydrogen ion**, which is acidic. The OH^- ion is the **hydroxide ion**, which is alkaline. Every water molecule (H_2O) that ionizes yields one hydrogen ion (H^+) and one hydroxide ion (OH^-). Therefore, in pure water, the concentration of acid and alkaline must be equal, since each time a hydrogen ion is produced, a hydroxide ion is also produced. In pure water, no other combinations are possible. This natural ionization of water explains two important ideas.

1. pH is only possible because of the ionization of water. Only aqueous (water) solutions have pH. Non-aqueous solutions (oil and alcohol) do not have pH. Without water, pH is not possible.

2. Pure water isn't neutral because it's neither acidic nor alkaline. Pure water is neutral because it's an even balance of both. Pure water is neutral because it contains the same number of hydrogen ions (H^+) as hydroxide ions (OH^-). Pure water is 50 percent acidic and 50 percent alkaline.

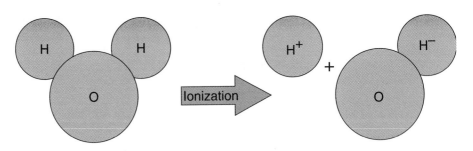

Figure 9-2 *The ionization of water into acid and alkali.*

THE pH SCALE

You may have heard the terms "parts hydrogen" or "potential hydrogen" used to describe the pH scale. Actually, the pH scale originates from the Danish term *potenz hydrogen* or "hydrogen strength" and was first proposed in 1909, by the Danish chemist S. P. L. Sorensen.

Scales are used to measure quantities. A ruler is a scale that is used to measure length. The **pH scale** measures acidity and alkalinity by measuring the concentration of hydrogen ions. The pH is the negative logarithm of the concentration of hydrogen ions. Notice that pH is written with a small "p" (which represents a quantity) and a capital "H". (which represents the hydrogen ion (H^+). The symbol pH represents the quantity of the hydrogen ion concentration.

Scientific notation is used to condense big numbers with many zeros. The number 1×10^{-7} is expressed in scientific notation and is the same number as .0000001, which is expressed as a decimal. Notice that in scientific notation the exponent is a seven. Also notice that the same number, expressed as a decimal, has seven decimal places. In scientific notation, a negative exponent is the same number as the number of decimal places and each decimal place indicates a ten-fold change. If we add a dollar sign to numbers expressed as a decimal, $0.01 is a penny (one cent) and $0.10 is a dime (ten cents). One penny times ten equals one dime. (See Fig. 9-3)

The term **logarithm** (LOG-ah-rhythm) means multiples of ten. Since the pH scale is a logarithmic scale, a change of one whole number represents a ten-fold change in pH. That means that a pH of 8 is ten times more alkaline than a pH of 7. A change of two whole numbers represents a change of ten times ten, or a one hundredfold change. That means that a pH of 9 is 100 times more alkaline than a pH of 7. A small change on the pH scale indicates a large change in the concentration of hydrogen and hydroxide ions.

The pH scale (Fig. 9-3) shows that the pH is simply the same number as the exponent, but without the minus sign. In scientific notation, the concentration of hydrogen ions in pure water is 1×10^{-7}. Notice that the exponent is seven, which is the pH of pure water. That means that the pH is the same number as the negative exponent in scientific notation. The pH of any solution is the exponent (of the hydrogen ion concentration) without the minus sign. Also notice that there is the same number of hydroxide ions (Fig. 9-3).

Regardless of pH, all aqueous solutions contain both acid (H^+) and alkaline (OH^-) ions. And although a pH of 6 is acidic, it is 10 times more alkaline than a pH of 5. Pure water, with a pH of 7, is 100 times more alkaline than a pH of 5. Since the average pH of hair and skin is also 5, pure water is 100 times more alkaline than your hair and skin, even though it has a neutral pH (Fig. 9-4). Pure water can cause the hair to swell as much as 20 percent.

Alkalinity increases as the pH increases and decreases as the pH decreases. That means that a higher pH (bigger number) is more alkaline than a lower pH

The pH Scale
H^+

pH	H^+ Hydrogen Ion		OH^- Hydroxide Ion	
	Exponential Notation	With Decimal	Exponential Notation	With Decimal
0	1×10^{-0}	1.	1×10^{-14}	.00000000000001
1	1×10^{-1}	.1	1×10^{-13}	.0000000000001
2	1×10^{-2}	.01	1×10^{-12}	.000000000001
3	1×10^{-3}	.001	1×10^{-11}	.00000000001
4	1×10^{-4}	.0001	1×10^{-10}	.0000000001
5	1×10^{-5}	.00001	1×10^{-9}	.000000001
6	1×10^{-6}	.000001	1×10^{-8}	.00000001
7	1×10^{-7}	.0000001	1×10^{-7}	.0000001
8	1×10^{-8}	.00000001	1×10^{-6}	.000001
9	1×10^{-9}	.000000001	1×10^{-5}	.00001
10	1×10^{-10}	.0000000001	1×10^{-4}	.0001
11	1×10^{-11}	.00000000001	1×10^{-3}	.001
12	1×10^{-12}	.000000000001	1×10^{-2}	.01
13	1×10^{-13}	.0000000000001	1×10^{-1}	.1
14	1×10^{-14}	.00000000000001	1×10^{-0}	1.

Figure 9-3 *The quantities of the pH scale expressed as pH, exponential notation, and with a decimal point.*

(smaller number). On the other hand, acidity increases as pH decreases. That means that a lower pH (smaller number) is more acidic than a higher pH (bigger number).

The pH scale only measures acidity (the hydrogen ion). The pH scale does not measure alkalinity (the hydroxide ion) directly, but it is understood because alkalinity increases as acidity decreases. Adding the exponents or decimal places across at any pH always totals 14 (Fig. 9-3).

ACIDS AND THE HYDROGEN ION (H^+)

All **acids** owe their chemical reactivity to the **hydrogen (HY-droh-jen) ion** (H^+). The word acid comes from the Latin acidus, meaning sour or tart. Acids contract and harden the hair (Fig. 9-4). Acids taste sour, turn litmus paper from blue to red, and react with akalis to form water and salts. Acids contract and harden the hair. Hydrochloric acid (HCl), commonly known as muratic acid, is a strong acid.

Solution	Effect on Hair		Important Features
Very Strong Acid (pH 0.0 – 1.0)	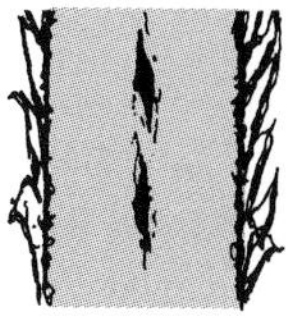	Dissolves hair completely.	Must not be applied to hair or scalp.
Strong to Mild Acid (pH 1.0 – 4.5)	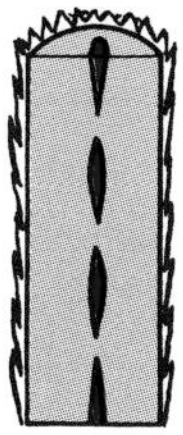	Hair shrinks and hardens. Body is increased. Cuticle imbrications close up. Porosity is reduced. Sheen of hair is improved. Soap residues are removed. Neutralizes traces of alkalies.	Acid or cream rinses restore body to bleached, porous hair. Conditioners and fillers overcome the excess porosity of damaged hair. Special shampoos reduce tangling and matting of hair and prevent color loss. Hair creams increase sheen. Color rinses provide temporary effect. Neutralizers remove residual waving lotion.
Neutral (pH 4.5 – 5.5)	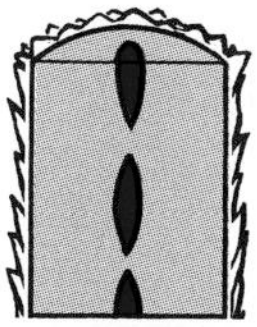	Hair is normal diameter. Texture and luster standard.	Neutral solutions are designed to prevent excess swelling of normal and damaged hair. Mild shampoos for normal cleaning and manageability of hair.
Mild Alkali (pH 5.5 – 10.0)	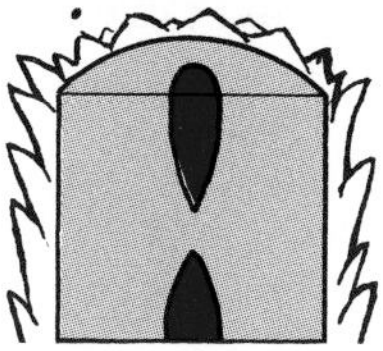	Hair swells. Porosity increases as imbrications open. Hair has a dry, drab appearance.	Tints and bleaches penetrate easier and chemical action increases. Cold wave solutions for resistant hair. Soap shampoos to overcome acidity of tap water. Activators for hydrogen peroxide.
Stronger Alkali (pH 10.0 – 14.0)	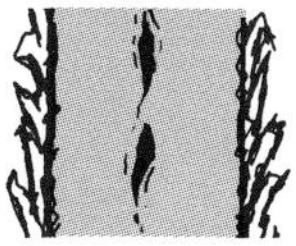	Dissolves hair completely	Must not be applied to hair or scalp unless used as relaxers or depilatories.

Figure 9-4 *The effect of pH on hair.*

Thioglyocolatic acid is used in permanent waving.

ALKALIS, BASES, AND THE HYDROXIDE ION (OH⁻)

All alkalis owe their chemical reactivity to the **hydroxide** (hy-DRAHKS-eyd) *ion* (OH^-). Although cosmetology still uses the term *alkali*, the scientific community usually uses the term *base*. The terms *alkali*, *alkaline*, *base*, and *basic* are interchangeable. Alkalis soften and swell the hair (Fig 9-4). Alkalis taste bitter, turn litmus paper from red to blue, feel slippery and soapy on the skin, and react with acids to form water and salts. Sodium hydroxide (NaOH), commonly known as lye, is a strong alkali used in chemical drain cleaners and chemical hair relaxers (see Chapter 14, Chemical Hair Relaxers and Soft Curl Permanents).

The Strengths of Acids and Alkalis

The hydrogen ion (H^+) is responsible for all acid reactions. The hydroxide ion (OH^-) is responsible for all alkaline reactions. The strength of different acids and alkalis is due to their degree of ionization in water. Strong acids and alkalis ionize almost completely and produce more ions. Weak acids and alkalis do not ionize completely and do not produce as many ions. Regardless of their strength, all acids produce hydrogen ions (H^+) and all alkalis produce hydroxide ions (OH^-). The only difference between strong acids and alkalis and weak acids and alkalis is the number of ions they produce.

Acid-Alkali Neutralization Reactions

When acids and alkalis are mixed together in equal proportions, they neutralize each other to form water and a salt. Although hydrochloric acid is a strong acid and sodium hydroxide is a strong alkali, if they are mixed together in exactly equal proportions, they form a solution of pure water and table salt. The neutralization reaction of hydrochloric acid (HCl) and sodium hydroxide (NaOH) to form salt water is shown below.

$$HCl + NaOH \rightarrow H_2O + NaCl$$

(or)

$$HCl + NaOH \rightarrow HOH + NaCl$$

OXIDATION-REDUCTION (REDOX) REACTIONS

The original discovery of **oxidation** reactions involved the chemical combination of any element or compound with oxygen to produce an oxide. When oxygen combines with another element, some heat is almost always produced. Chemical reactions that produce heat are called **exothermic** ("exo" means outside and "thermic" means heat). Exothermic permanent waves produce heat because of an oxidation reaction that results when the activator tube, which contains hydrogen peroxide, is added to the permanent wave solution (see Chapter 13, Permanent Waving).

Slow oxidation occurs in oxidation haircolors and permanent wave neutralizers. If you pay close attention, you will notice an increase in the temperature of oxidation haircolors after the peroxide is added. *Combustion* is a *rapid oxidation* reaction that produces a high quantity of heat and light. Lighting a match is an example of rapid oxidation. Remember, you can't have a fire without oxygen.

When oxygen is combined with a substance, the substance is oxidized. When oxygen is removed from a substance, the substance is **reduced**. Oxidizing agents are substances that readily release oxygen. Hydrogen peroxide is an oxidizing agent because it contains "extra" oxygen. When hydrogen peroxide is mixed with an oxidation haircolor, the haircolor gains oxygen and is oxidized. At the same time, the hydrogen peroxide loses oxygen and the hydrogen peroxide is reduced. In this example, haircolor is the reducing agent.

Oxidation and reduction always occur simultaneously and are referred to as *redox* reactions. Oxidation cannot happen without reduction. In a redox reaction, the oxidizer is always reduced and the reducing agent is always oxidized.

So far, we have considered oxidation only as the addition of oxygen, and reduction only as the loss of oxygen. Although the first known oxidation reactions involved oxygen, many oxidation reactions do not involve oxygen. Oxidation also results from the loss of hydrogen, and reduction also results from the addition of hydrogen.

Permanent waving is an example of this type of redox reaction. Permanent waving solution contains thioglycolic acid. Permanent wave solution breaks the disulfide bonds in the hair through a reduction reaction that adds hydrogen ions (H^+) to the hair. In this reaction, the hair is reduced and the perm solution is oxidized. Neutralizer then oxidizes the hair by removing the hydrogen that was previously added. When the hair is oxidized, the neutralizer is reduced (see Chapter 13, Permanent Waving).

For our purposes, **oxidation** can be defined as either the addition of oxygen or the loss of hydrogen. Conversely, **reduction** can be defined as either the loss of oxygen or the addition of hydrogen.

REVIEW QUESTIONS

1. Define pH.

2. How much more acidic is pH 2 than pH 6?

3. What is the pH of an organic solvent that is insoluble in water?

4. Which is most dangerous to the skin or eyes: acids, bases, or corrosives? Why?

5. What is the importance of the skin's acid mantle?

6. What safety precautions should you take when using oxidizers?

Discussion Questions

1. Ask your instructor about the importance placed on safety when she or he attended cosmetology school. Is more importance placed on safety today than there was ten years ago?

Chapter 10

Shampoos, Conditioners, and Styling Aids

Key Terms

Amphoteric surfactants
Anionic surfactants
Cationic surfactants
Chlorofluorocarbons
Detergent
Emulsions
Fatty alcohols
Fatty materials
Hydrogen bonding
Hydrophilic
Hydrophobic
Inverse micelles
Lipophilic
Lipophobic
micelle
Nonionic surfactants
Oil-in-water emulsions
SD (alcohol)
Silicones
Soaps
Surface tension
Surfactant
Volatile alcohols
Volatile organic compounds
Water-in-oil emulstions

Learning Objectives

After completing this chapter, you should be able to:

- Understand and explain the chemistry of shampoo.

- Describe the relationship among soaps, detergents, and surfactants.

- Explain how wetting improves product performance and chemical services.

- List the basic types of surfactants.

- Define ions.

- Understand folklore chemicals and why they are used.

- Describe the purpose for each ingredient in shampoos and conditioners.

- Understand hydrogen bonding and surface tension.

INTRODUCTION

Shampoos, conditioners and styling aids are emulsions. **Emulsions** (ee-MUL-shuns) are mixtures of two immiscible liquids (usually oil and water) dispersed by an emulsifying agent. The term *emulsify* means "to form an emulsion," which is a mixture of one liquid dispersed in another (Chapter 8, General Chemistry). Since water is the major ingredient in most of the emulsions a hairstylist uses, let's begin our study of emulsions by examining the properties of water that are essential to understanding emulsions.

WATER IS POLAR

The earth is *polar*, which means it has both a north and a south pole with opposite magnetic charges. Water is also polar, which means it has opposite electrical charges at opposite ends of its molecule (Figs. 10-1 and 10-2). The hydrogen end

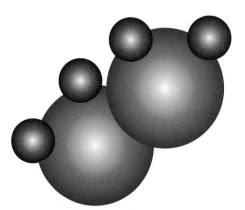

Figure 10-1 *Three dimensional representation of water molecules.*
(Reprinted with permission of Padi Americas)

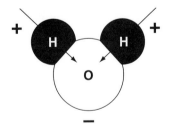

Figure 10-2 *Water molecule showing a positive charge on the hydrogen end and a negative charge on the oxygen end.*
(Reprinted with permission of Padi Americas)

of a water molecule has a slight positive charge and the oxygen end of a water molecule has a slight negative charge.

Hydrogen Bonding and Surface Tension

Since opposites attract, the positive (hydrogen) end of one water molecule is attracted to the negative (oxygen) end of another water molecule. This attraction between water molecules is a special type of ionic bonding called **hydrogen bonding** (Figure 10-3). Hydrogen bonding is like "sticky glue" that holds water molecules together. This attraction between water molecules is called **surface tension**. Surface tension tends to minimize the surface area and acts like a flexible skin on the surface of water. Surface tension permits insects to "walk" on the surface of water and causes water to be shaped in a spherical drop (Figure 10-4).

Water has the ability to dissolve many polar substances because of its polar nature. Since "like dissolves like," water acts as a solvent for most other ionic substances, as well as those that have the ability to hydrogen bond. Substances that dissolve in water are **hydrophilic** (hy-droh-**FIL**-ik), which means water loving, from "hydro" (water) and "philic" (love).

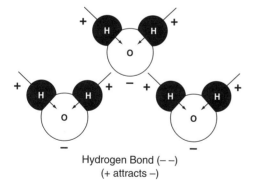

Hydrogen Bond (– –)
(+ attracts –)

Figure 10-3 *Water molecules showing hydrogen bonding due to opposite electrical charges on the water molecules.*
(Reprinted with permission of Padi Americas)

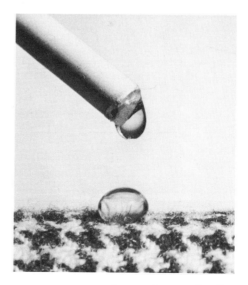

Figure 10-4 *Drops of water showing the effects of surface tension and the lack of "wetting".*
(Courtesy: Unilever Ltd.)

OILS ARE NONPOLAR

Oils are nonpolar, have no electric charge and do not hydrogen bond. Oils mix with oils, but do not mix with water. Oils are **lipophilic** (lip-oh-**FIL**-ik), which means oil loving, from "lipid" (oil) and "philic" (love). Although water is called the universal solvent, it can't dissolve oils. You have probably heard the saying, "oil and water don't mix."

Not only do oil and water not mix, water actually repels oil because of hydrogen bonding and surface tension. So in addition to water being hydrophilic (water loving), water is also **lipophobic** (lip-oh-**FOH**-bik), which means oil hating, from "lipid" (oil) and "phobic" (hating). Conversely, oil is lipophilic (oil loving) and is also **hydrophobic** (hy-droh-**FOH**-bik), which means water hating, from "hydro" (water) and "phobic" (hating).

SURFACTANTS

Now that we know why oil and water don't mix, let's see how surfactants overcome those obstacles to form an emulsion. The name **surfactant** (sur-**FAK**-tant) is a contraction for surface active agent (**surf**ace **act**ive age**nt**). Surfactants are able to wet the hair and disperse oil in water by reducing surface tension. A surfactant molecule has two distinct parts that make the emulsification of oil and water possible (Fig. 10-5). One end of the surfactant molecule is hydrophilic (water loving) and the other end is lipophilic (oil loving). Since "like dissolves like," the hydrophilic end dissolves in water and the lipophilic end dissolves in oil. So, a surfactant molecule dissolves in both oil and water and joins them together.

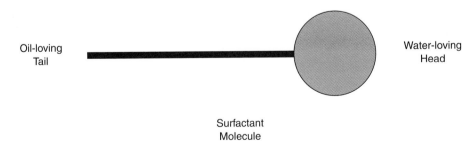

Oil-loving
Tail

Water-loving
Head

Surfactant
Molecule

Figure 10-5 *Surfactant molecule showing an oil-loving tail and a water-loving head.*

SHAMPOO

Shampoo sinks aren't the most glamorous spot in the salon, but that's where a lot of the action is. The success or failure of many chemical services depends on using the proper shampoo.

Proper shampooing and conditioning are among the most important services performed in the salon. Too often clients are passed quickly through this essential process. Proper cleansing of the hair is vital and should not be underestimated.

Imagine allowing three or four minutes to cleanse and thoroughly rinse 100,000 individual hair fibers with over 40 square feet of hair on the average head.

Thanks to surfactants, a marvel of modern chemistry, the hair and scalp can be gently and safely cleansed.

SHAMPOO CHEMISTRY

Oils, such as sebum, are insoluble in water. Sebum combines with dead cells from the scalp, dust, pollen, smoke, and other environmental contaminants to form a sticky, oily coating on the hair and scalp. It is difficult to remove oils or other water-insoluble substances from the hair. It is much like trying to rinse Vaseline from a cashmere sweater (Figs. 10-6–10-8).

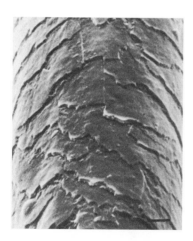

Figure 10-6 *Normal clean hair, magnified 5,000 times.*
(Courtesy: *Gillette Company Research Institute,* Rockville, Maryland)

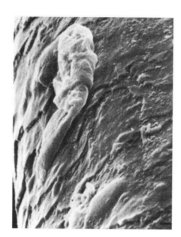

Figure 10-7 *Normal hair with accumulated sebum and debis, magnified 7,500 times.*
(Courtesy: *Gillette Company Research Institute,* Rockville, Maryland)

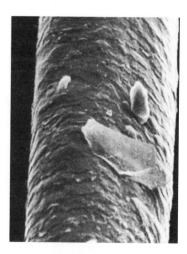

Figure 10-8 *Normal hair with dandruff flakes adhering to fiber, magnified 1,200 times.*
(Courtesy: *Gillette Company Research Institute,* Rockville, Maryland)

Soaps

Detergent is a Latin word for a "wiping-off substance." **Soaps** are the most common types of detergents. Records of their use date back 5,000 years to the ancient Babylonians. Soaps are made by mixing plant oils or animal fat with strong alkaline (basic) substances. Typically, coconut oil, palm oil, castor oil, and/or olive oil are used in soaps.

Soaps have several disadvantages. They combine with hard water to form stubborn, insoluble films. These films coat and dull the hair. Also, the high alkalinity of soap has a negative effect on hair and skin. Small amounts of soap are still used in modern shampoos but only as thickeners or to give a pearlescent look.

Surfactants

These unique molecules prove that "natural" is not always better. In fact, chemistry often provides great improvements upon nature. Surfactants are designed to be mild and easily rinsed from the hair.

Surfactants work by getting between the surface of the oil and water. Surfactants are happiest when they are at the oil and water interface (the boundary where oil meets water). They flood into the interface and concentrate there (Figs. 10-9–10-12).

The "water-loving," hydrophilic head penetrates into the water portion of the interface. At the same time, the "oil-loving," lipophilic tail pokes in the oily substances on the hair. The result is that the oil makes a bead and floats off the hair shaft (Figs. 10-13–10-17).

This bead of oil is completely surrounded by surfactant molecules that form a sphere called a **micelle** (**MY**-cell) (Figure 10-20). Thanks to the surfactant, this

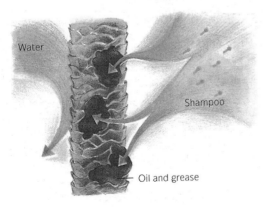

Figure 10-9 *Tail of shampoo molecules is attracted to hair, grease, and dirt.*

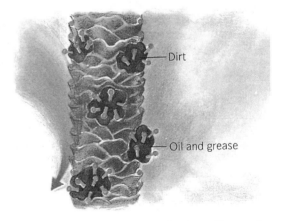

Figure 10-10 *Surfactant molecules collect at the oil/water interface, causing the oil to form a bead.*

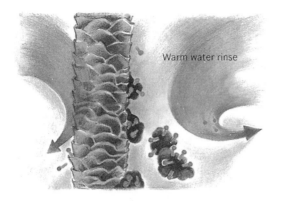

Figure 10-11 *Rinsing with water dislodges the beads of oil and debris from the hair shaft.*

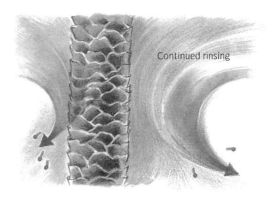

Figure 10-12 *Continued rinsing is necessary to remove remaining surfactant molecules.*

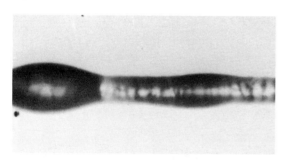

Figure 10-13 *Oil coated hair.*
(*Courtesy: British Launderers Research Association*)

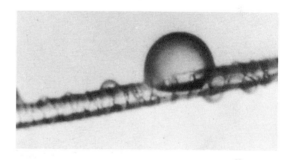

Figure 10-14 *Oil bead is starting to form.*
(*Courtesy: Dr. J A. Kichener, Royal College of Science*)

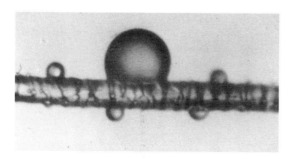

Figure 10-15 *Bead has less contact with the surface of the hair shaft.*

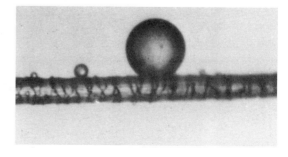

Figure 10-16 *Oil bead is barely touching the hair shaft.*

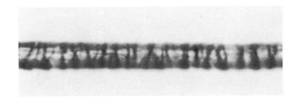

Figure 10-17 *Oil floats away, leaving hair clean.*

droplet of oil is now emulsified (dispersed) in water, within the micelle, until more water can rinse it away. When the hair is rinsed, the emulsified oil and dirt that are bound to the water are carried away with it.

Gentle massaging of the scalp and hair is important. Massaging helps the surfactant remove the oily emulsions. This process, along with the proper wetting techniques, allow the product to penetrate the hair shaft and work more efficiently (Fig. 10-18).

We have all seen shampoo advertisements showing happy, beautiful people taking showers with their heads heaped high with mounds of lather. These images have taught the public to associate lather with cleansing ability. The truth is, lots of foamy lather only means too much shampoo is used. Excess foam equals waste!

Sebum and other oils quickly destroy foam. Ideally, the head should have just enough lather to lubricate the scalp and hair. This will help your fingers massage the shampoo more effectively into the hair.

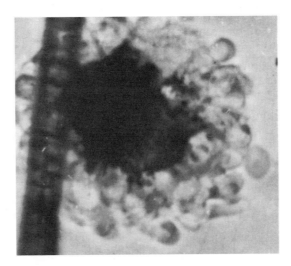

Figure 10-18 *The action of a shampoo on dirt particles attached to a fiber. The surfactant molecules surround the dirt and help to lever it off with the aid of proper rinsing.*
(Courtesy: British Launderers Research Association)

LATHER UP!

People expect a lot from shampoos. Unfortunately, it isn't always easy to tell a good shampoo from a poor one. Cost, fragrance, and lots of foam is what most people look for in shampoo.

Lather or foam is of little importance, but it often gets the most attention. Foaming occurs when surfactant molecules gather around air instead of oil. The result is millions of tiny bubbles. Obviously, the air bubbles are using the surfactants that should be removing dirt and oil (Figure 10–19).

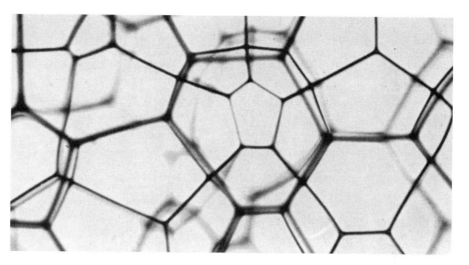

Figure 10–19 A *magnified view of foam bubbles.*
(Courtesy: Dr. J. A. Kichener, Royal College of Science)

Fragrances and foaming qualities are not good ways to evaluate shampoos. Examine the hair condition after several uses. Is it flyaway, is it hard to comb, does it seem limp, do the colors fade, is the hair dry or the scalp itchy?

Carefully choose the shampoo to use and recommend. The quality of your services and the success of your repeat business may depend on the decision of product choice.

All surfactants aren't detergents. Many surfactants do not clean well enough to be used as a detergent but are still essential to the formation of emulsions. Different surfactants perform different functions and serve many purposes. Surfactants are used as detergents, wetting agents, emulsifiers, stabilizers, foam builders, conditioners, thickeners, and pearling agents. All soaps and detergents are surfactants, but all surfactants aren't soaps or detergents.

Emulsions

An **emulsion** is a mixture of one liquid dispersed in another. One of the liquids is usually oil and the other is usually water. These two immiscible liquids form two distinct phases. The two most common types of emulsions are oil-in-water (O/W) and water-in-oil (W/O).

Oil-in-Water (O/W) Emulsions

In **oil-in-water emulsions,** droplets of oil are dispersed in water. The droplets of oil (micelles) are surrounded by surfactants with their "tails" (lipophilic ends) pointing in and their "heads" (hydrophilic ends) pointing out, which keeps the oil dispersed in water (Fig. 10-21). In O/W emulsions, the water is the continuous or external phase and the oil is discontinuous or internal phase (Figure 10-

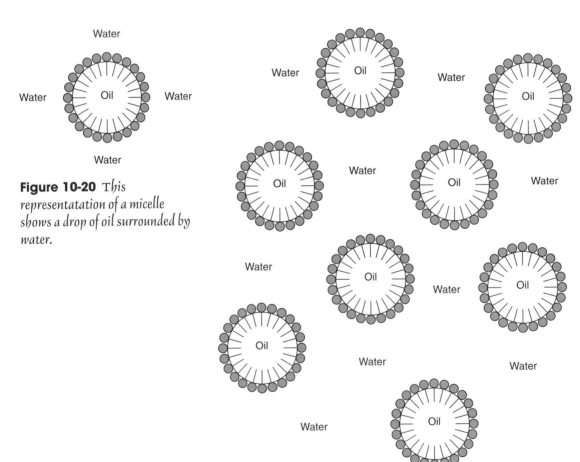

Figure 10-20 *This representatation of a micelle shows a drop of oil surrounded by water.*

Figure 10-21 *Many micelles form an oil-in-water emulsion with droplets of oil suspended in water. Oil is the internal phase and water is the external phase.*

21). Oil-in-water emulsions usually contain a small amount of oil and a greater amount of water. Most of the emulsions used in a salon are oil-in-water.

Water-in-Oil (W/O) Emulsions

In a **water-in-oil emulsion**, droplets of water are dispersed in oil. The droplets of water (**inverse micelles**) are surrounded by surfactants with their "heads" (hydrophilic ends) pointing in and their "tails" (lipophilic ends) pointing out. (Fig. 10-22). In W/O emulsions, the oil is the continuous or external phase and the water is discontinuous, or internal phase (Figure 10.23). Water-in-oil emulsions usually contain a smaller amount of water and a greater amount of oil. Cold creams are water-in-oil emulsions.

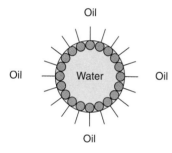

Figure 10-22 *This representation of an inverse micelle shows a droplet of water surrounded by oil.*

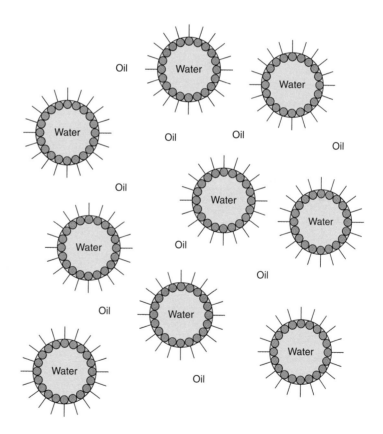

Figure 10-23 *Many inverse micelles from a water-in-oil emulsion with droplets of water suspended in oil. Water is the internal phase and oil is the external phase.*

Multiple Phase (W/O/W) Emulsions

Multiple phase emulsions have more than two phases. In a water-in-oil-in-water (W/O/W) emulsion, a two-phase W/O emulsion is dispersed in water. Multiple phase emulsions are able to encapsulate active ingredients to reduce skin irritation and provide longer shelf life. On dilution during rinsing, encapsulated particles break apart and deposit active ingredients on the hair and skin.

Microemulsions

Microemulsions have a small micelle size. Standard emulsions, without adding coloring, are usually white because of the refraction of light by the micelles, but microemulsions are transparent because their micelles are too small to be "seen" by light. The white, titanium dioxide sunblock usually worn by lifeguards, can now be completely transparent because of the technology of microemulsions.

Liposomes

Liposomes (**LYE**-poh-sohmes) are water compartments (vesicles) enclosed by a lipid bilayer (two-layer micelles). These two single layers have their hydrophobic "tails" facing each other and their hydrophilic "heads" facing the water. This structure is similar to the cell membrane that encloses all the cells of the body. Like microemulsions, liposomes have the ability to separate active ingredients, which keeps them stable and aids in the delivery of active ingredients.

The major types of surfactants are:

Anionic (an-eye-**ON**-ick)

Cationic (kat-eye-**ON**-ick)

Nonionic (non-eye-**ON**-ick)

Amphoteric (am-fo-**TERR**-ick)

Anionic Surfactants (Negatively Charged)

Anionic surfactants are the most widely used detergents in the cosmetology profession. They are inexpensive, simple to prepare, and excellent cleaners. They also rinse easily from the hair. A major disadvantage is that they can be harsh and irritating to the scalp. Frequently, other surfactants and ingredients are added to reduce skin irritation.

Cationic Surfactants (Positively Charged)

Cationic surfactants are rarely used in high concentrations in the cosmetology profession. Many types are dangerous to the eyes, but are safe and useful in low amounts. Until recently, their positive charges prevented them from being mixed with negatively charged anionic surfactants. Newer types, however, eliminate this incompatibility.

Cationic surfactants are antibacterial. Because of their positive charge, they form ionic bonds (salt bonds) with the negatively charged surface of the hair. (Hair has a multitude of ionic bonds. The negative ions outnumber the positive; therefore, the surface of the hair carries a negative charge.) The result is better wet combing, softness, and gloss. The most important cationic surfactants are quaternary ammonium compounds, referred to as "quats." Quats are substantive (resist being rinsed away) because of their positive charge that attracts and bonds them to negatively charged hair. Quats are excellent conditioners that improve wet combing, reduce static electricity, and improve flyaway hair.

Nonionic Surfactants (No Charge)

Nonionic surfactants have neither a positive nor a negative charge. Once again, the name tells you something about the nature of these chemicals. By themselves, they are not useful as cleansing agents, but nonionic surfactants are found in

SAPONINS—NATURE'S SURFACTANTS

Saponins (**SAP**-uh-nins) are an unusual set of nonionic surfactants. Saponins are called natural surfactants because they are the only ones found in nature. Plants like soapbark, soapwort, sarsaparilla, and ivy contain large amounts of this chemical.

Sound pretty wonderful, don't they? The interesting thing about saponins is that they are terrible surfactants. Saponins proved to be such poor cleansing and conditioning agents, they were not used for many years. Even though these natural surfactants are useless, the craze for natural ingredients has caused some manufacturers to include them in shampoo products.

This is just one example of a *folklore ingredient*. Many shampoos contain folklore ingredients. Folklore is defined as traditions or beliefs passed on by word of mouth. These beliefs are not based on scientific fact. Sometimes, science can verify the belief, but usually, they are proven untrue.

Many natural ingredients used in shampoos and conditioners are folklore chemicals. Generally, there is no scientific evidence to back up the claims made for these ingredients.

For example, the ancients believed that rosemary oil strengthened the memory and kept lovers faithful. Modern wisdom says that it enhances the highlights and stimulates hair growth. The truth is rosemary oil is a toxic skin and eye irritant.

The public incorrectly assumes anything "natural" must be good. Names like cucumber juice, nettle, or goldenrod extract dupe a consumer into paying more for insignificant amounts of fancy-sounding herbs or botanical extracts.

Don't buy a product just because it has exotic-sounding ingredients. Buy a product because it works better.

nearly all shampoo formulations. Usually, they are added to make anionic surfactants milder and less irritating.

Amphoteric Surfactants (Positively or Negatively Charged)

The charge on an **amphoteric surfactant** depends entirely upon the shampoo's pH level. At low pHs (less than 5 or 6), they are positively charged, like cationic surfactants. At higher pHs, they become negatively charged, like anionic surfactants. In between the high and low pH value, they have no charge, like nonionic surfactants.

This versatility makes amphoteric surfactants extremely useful. They have the conditioning properties of cationic surfactants but have a lower skin sensitivity and eye irritation. These surfactants are often found in nonstinging or baby shampoos. They are more costly than anionic surfactants and don't cleanse as well, but they make excellent additions to high-quality shampoos.

Ethoxylated Surfactants

Ethoxylates are formed by the addition of ethylene oxide to a fatty material. **Ethoxylated surfactants** decrease skin and eye irritation and increases solubility. Sodium laureth sulfate is an ethoxylated version of sodium lauryl sulfate. Other common ethoxylates are octoxynol-40, nonoxynol-10 and polysorbate 80.

Typical Shampoo Formulations

Water

Shampoos in gel, cream, or liquid states need large amounts of water to keep all of the ingredients dissolved. Water is the solvent in shampoo. Typically, between 45 and 75 percent of the content is water.

Surfactants

Surfactants make up between 30 and 40 percent of a shampoo's content. As mentioned previously, it is common to use blends of three or four different surfactants.

Foam Builders and Stabilizers

The purpose for adding foam builders and stabilizers is to create large amounts of thick, creamy-feeling bubbles. Although the effect is only cosmetic, small amounts of foam do help a person spread the shampoo through the hair.

Antistatic Detanglers

Detanglers are usually low concentrations of cationic surfactants that coat the hair shaft and improve wet combing. They also reduce static and flyaway hair.

Thickeners

Thickeners help control the final thickness of the shampoo. With so much water content, shampoos would be thin without thickeners. The major types of thickeners used are plant gums and synthetic polymers. Thickeners are also used to make gels. These additives prevent ingredients from settling to the bottom of the bottle.

Conditioners

Conditioners are the ingredients that add shine, gloss, and emollience to the hair. Some also act as moisturizers.

Chelators (Sequestrants)

Chelate (**KEE**-late) means "claw" in Latin. The chemical structure of chelators have clawlike branches. The claw grabs and holds the calcium or magnesium ions found in water. These ions are the reason for hard water. The more of these ions found in the water, the harder the water. Calcium and magnesium ions cause soap film (the deposits on shower walls and bath tubs). Chelators prevent films from depositing on the hair shaft.

Opacifiers and Pearling Agents

The disadvantage of clear shampoos is that many useful additives can't be used. They would cloud the product or make it look unattractive. Cremes and opaque products offer the widest range of possibilities. Formulators are less restricted and can add an extensive variety of ingredients. *Opacifiers* cover up cloudiness or unattractive colors. *Pearling agents* give a "pearlescent" texture to shampoos.

Preservatives

Many shampoo and conditioner ingredients provide a source of food for mold or bacteria. *Preservatives* inhibit their growth and improve the shampoo's shelf life. Without preservatives, shampoos would not be as safe. For example, certain types of bacteria produce toxins that damage the eyes or can cause blindness.

Some individuals develop allergic sensitivities to preservatives, but the advantages of preservatives far outweigh any occasional problems. Thanks to preservatives and the care taken by manufacturers, shampoos and conditioners are some of the safest cosmetic products available. If reactions or other problems occur, consult the shampoo Material Safety Data Sheet (MSDS) and refer to a dermatologist.

Fragrances and Coloring

Fragrance and coloring make up less than one percent of the shampoo formula but are responsible for over 90 percent of shampoo sales. Neither ingredient is necessary or useful beyond improving appearance and odor. Never choose a shampoo simply because it smells good or has a pretty color.

Common Shampoo Ingredients

Shampoos are oil-in-water emulsions designed to clean hair and skin with minimum damage and irritation. Some of the more common ingredients are listed in the table below along with their function. Many ingredients have dozens of minor variations, far too many to list here. Sodium sulfate/ammonium sulfate, lauryl sulfate/laureth sulfate, and cocamide MEA/cocamide DEA are examples of similar ingredients with similar names.

The only way to learn about the products you use is to read the back of the bottle. Although at first it may seem impossible, it doesn't take long to learn to recognize the most common ingredients. Once you can identify the top ten, you will be amazed at how similar many of the products you use really are. Shampoos, liquid hand soaps, and bubble baths all clean hair and skin and contain many of the same ingredients. Lists of product ingredients can be found in Appendix F.

Function	Ingredient
Diluent	Water
Primary Surfactants (Detergents)	Sodium Lauryl Sulfate, Ammonium Laureth Sulfate TEA Sulfate
Secondary Surfactants	Cocamidopropyl Betaine, Lauryl Polyglucose, Sulfosuccinate, Isethionate, Hydroxysultaine
Foam Stabilizers	Cocamide DEA, Lauramide DEA
Viscosity Builders	Sodium Chloride, Ammonium Chloride
Pearling Agents/ Opacifiers	Glycol Distearate,
Thickener/Stabilizer	Hydroxyethyl Cellulose, Gum Arabic, Acacia, Sodium Algenate, Carrageenan, Chitin, Guar, Xanthan, Vegum, Carbomer 940, Silicates, PEG
Preservative	Methylparaben, Propylparaben, Methylisothiazolinone,
Sequestrant/Chelator	EDTA, Sodium Citrate, Trisodium Phosphate
Anti-Dandruff	Zinc Pyrithione, Salicylic Acid, Sulfur, Coal Tar, Menthol

CONDITIONER CHEMISTRY

Surfactants are better than soap but still aren't perfect. They can't remove only the dirty oil and leave the oils essential for healthy hair. Since daily shampooing may cause excessively dry hair, regular conditioning will help the hair regain much of its lost shine and body.

Other factors influence the condition of the hair and scalp. Chemical damage results from permanent wave lotion, excessive bleaching, peroxide, color, blow dryers, medicated shampoos, and exposure to weather. Air pollutants, wind, sea, and chlorinated pool water also can cause damage to the hair shaft.

Sunlight is very damaging and causes significant damage to the hair, even to virgin hair. Damaged hair looks lifeless and dull. It breaks more easily, is more porous, and dries more slowly.

It is optimistic to believe that any conditioner will repair damaged hair. The best we can hope for is to restore hair's natural appearance and feel. The hard keratin surface of hair is a tight mesh of cuticles. The outer layers are very *hydrophobic*, especially on virgin hair. This prevents most conditioning agents from deeply penetrating the hair shaft. In most cases, a conditioning agent merely coats and lubricates the outer hair shaft. This causes consumers to believe the hair is healthier, when actually it only has a slippery-feeling texture.

Little can be done to truly improve the condition of virgin hair. However, damaged hair is more porous and absorbs larger amounts of conditioning chemicals.

This does not mean that conditioners are unnecessary or useless. They can significantly improve the appearance and manageability of hair. A well-formulated conditioner can improve the hair's life, volume, spring, sheen, softness, and manageability, and reduce static flyaway. However, it is important to realize that these improvements do not mean the hair has been restored to its original health.

Conditioning shampoos have some value but are limited in performance. Adding heavy or deep conditioning agents to shampoo interferes with the action of the shampoo and actually traps debris on the hair shaft (Fig. 10-24).

Dry-formula shampoos contain moisture-attracting chemicals that increase the water content of damaged hair. Fine/limp hair shampoos frequently depend on polymers or other materials that coat the hair with a thin film. These films add body and bounce, however, they may build up with repeated use.

Since we've already learned so much about shampoo ingredients, learning about conditioners will be easy. Hair conditioners can really be thought of as

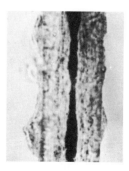

Figure 10-24 *Hair soiled with excess hair cream, which must be removed by shampoo.*

inverted shampoos. Most shampoos contain a large amount of surfactant and a small amount of fatty material (conditioner). On the other hand, most hair conditioners contain a large amount of fatty material (conditioner) and a small amount of surfactant. Yes, conditioners contain surfactants, often the same ones used in shampoos. Without surfactants, conditioners wouldn't lather and couldn't be rinsed from the hair.

In addition to the surfactants already discussed in shampoos, a well-designed conditioner contains the following types of ingredients:

Protein and Protein Derivatives

Since proteins are long chains containing hundreds of amino acids, it is nearly impossible for them to penetrate the hair shaft. There is some chance that damaged, porous hair will absorb useful amounts of protein, but damaged hair cannot be reconstructed from additives. Some studies indicate that small proteins help seal split ends and prevent them from getting worse. In general, the smaller the protein and the greater hair damage, the more absorption.

Concentrated protein conditioners are used to increase the tensile strength of the hair and to temporarily close split ends. These conditioners use hydrolized protein (small fragments) and are designed to pass through the cuticle, penetrate into the cortex, and replace the keratin that has been lost from the hair. They improve texture, equalize porosity, and increase elasticity.

Fatty Materials

Hair conditioners improve wet combing and make hair feel soft by depositing **fatty materials** on the hair. Fatty materials are the backbone of many conditioners. Most conditioners contain large amounts of several different types of fatty materials.

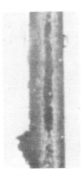

Figure 10-25 Hair with attached dirt particles, dandruff scales, sebum coating.

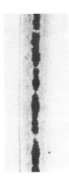

Figure 10-26 Same hair after cleaning with a mildly acid soapless shampoo.

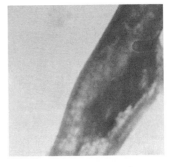

Figure 10-27 Hair after continued washing with highly alkaline soap. Note swelling and severe damage to shaft.

Fatty Alcohols

When most consumers think of alcohol, they think only of small, light-weight, volatile alcohols like methyl alcohol (wood alcohol), isopropyl alcohol (rubbing alcohol), and ethyl alcohol (alcoholic beverages). But those aren't the only kinds of alcohols. **Fatty alcohols** are large, non-volatile oils, fats or waxes, which contain an alcohol group, and are used as conditioners. Cetyl alcohol, cetearyl alcohol, stearyl alcohol, and myristyl alcohol are some of the most common fatty alcohols.

Silicones

Silicones (SIL-ih-kohnz) are oils that contain a repeating silicon-oxygen chain. Silicones belong to a family of chemicals called polysiloxanes. Silicones are superior to their plain oil counterparts because they are less greasy and form a "breathable" film that is non-comedogenic. Amodimethicone, cyclomethicone and dimethicone are examples of silicon conditioners.

Humectants

Unique chemicals called *humectants* absorb water and hold it tightly. Humectants are used to keep many products from drying out. They are also used in skin and hair care products, i.e., damaged or dry hair shampoos. Humectants act like microscopic sponges, attracting moisture to the skin and hair. Common humectants such as sodium PCA, sodium lactate, and glycerin, are found in conditioners.

Moisturizers

The term *moisturizer* is applied freely to many ingredients. Since only water can moisturize, it is a misleading name for substances other than water. Frequently, moisturizers refer to oily substances (not water soluble) that coat the hair (or skin), preventing water loss by evaporation. Lanolin, mineral oil, and cholesterol are examples of water-trapping additives found in many conditioners and other types of cosmetic products.

Naturals, Botanicals and Vitamins

Many consumers believe that botanical ingredients are healthier, more natural and more effective, even though there is no scientific evidence to support those claims. There is no formal definition of the term "natural." And natural does not always mean better or safer. Poison ivy is natural, but I wouldn't want it in my shampoo. Natural gas is a colorless, odorless, toxic gas. The pungent odor associated with natural gas is added as a warning, so that its presence can be detected. Even chemicals that have no smell may not be safe.

Essence of chamomile, rose hips, and yarrow may sound great, but in reality these are solutions of mostly water. There is no scientific evidence to indicate that botanical ingredients are any more effective than chemicals from other sources. Botanicals are processed and preserved and contain solvents, diluents, and other unknown ingredients that may not even be listed on the product label.

According to Donald A. Davis, the editor of *Drug and Cosmetic Industry Magazine*, "By their very nature, cosmetics have to build upon the expectations, dreams and wish fulfillment of those who buy and use them. The gap between what is promised and what is really attainable unduly abuses credibility. They throw into disrepute some serious technological advances now being made in an industry that was too long noted for the shallowness of its scientific curiosity about the workings of the skin and hair."

Styling Aids

The two main types of styling aids are setting lotions (gels) and hairsprays. Both setting lotions and hairsprays hold hair in place by depositing a flexible film of polymeric resins. Setting lotions are usually applied to wet hair and then dried, while hairsprays are usually applied to dry hair after styling.

A good styling lotion should increase body and volume and improve hold. It should also comb easily, not be sticky, be quick drying, and not flake when brushed. Since most modern styling lotions are emulsions, many of the ingredients are the same ones found in shampoos and conditioners. The main ingredients in setting lotions are polymeric resins, thickeners, nonionic surfactants, fragrances, preservatives and sometimes alcohol.

Conditioning gels and leave-in conditioners have the same basic formula, but the polymeric resin is usually replaced with a cationic conditioning polymer. Protein derivatives and quats may also be added as conditioning agents.

Polymeric Resins

The most important ingredient in any setting lotion is the *polymeric resin* that provides the hold. The amount of resin used affects the degree of holding power. A higher concentration of resin forms a harder film and firmer hold. The main hair fixative polymers commonly used in setting lotions are: Polyvinylpyrrolidone (PVP), Polyquaternium, PVM/MA Copolymer, and Octylacrylamide/Acrylates.

Nonionic Surfactants

Most setting lotions are emulsions and nonionic surfactants used as emulsifiers. Nonionic surfactants may also soften the resin and provide some conditioning. Examples include Laureth-23, Oleth-20, and Steareth-20.

Alcohols

Although fatty alcohols may be used in some styling lotions for conditioning, **volatile alcohols** are often added to shorten the drying time and increase hold.

Many hairstylists apply hairspray to a roller set to speed-up drying. SD Alcohol is by far the most common volatile alcohol used in setting lotions.

SD (specially denatured) alcohol is ethyl alcohol or ethanol and is the same alcohol found in alcoholic beverages. SD stands for specially denatured. Denaturants are added to ethyl alcohol to make it unsuitable for human consumption. Denaturants have an intensely bitter taste that renders the alcohol unpalatable. Denatured alcohol is not subject to the consumption tax that must be paid if ethyl alcohol is used as a beverage. Although alcohol-free setting lotions are thought to be less drying to the hair, that's not necessarily true. Any dryness caused by alcohol is reversed as soon as the hair is wet.

Hairsprays

Setting lotions are usually applied to wet hair and then dried, while hairsprays are usually applied to dry hair, either as the style is being finished or after the styling has been completed. Setting lotions are mostly water and need not contain any volatile organic compounds. Hairsprays, on the other hand, must contain a majority of volatile organic compounds and a minimum of water, as too much water would wet the hair and ruin the finished hairstyle.

Although there are some variations, the resins used in hairsprays and setting lotions are much the same. The major difference between setting lotions and hairsprays is the amount of water that is used. Hairsprays rely on the use of volatile organic compounds (VOCs) with little water.

Volatile Organic Compounds (VOCs)

The name **volatile organic compounds** (VOCs) describe exactly what these chemicals are. VOCs are two or more elements combined chemically (compounds) that contain carbon (organic) and evaporate quickly (volatile).

Although smog is not a problem in sparsely populated areas, it has become a large problem in cities like Los Angeles. Even though automobile exhaust is the major cause of photochemical smog, VOCs also contribute. In the early '90s, the Environmental Protection Agency (EPA) required the reduction of all VOCs in hairsprays to be less than 80 percent. It should come as no surprise that California regulations are more restrictive. The California Air Resource Board (CARB) now restricts the VOCs in hairsprays to be less than 55 percent. Many manufactures now make the same hairspray in two different formulas, one for California (55 percent) and another (80 percent) for the rest of the United States.

Pump and Aerosol Hairsprays

The most common VOC used in pump hairsprays is SD Alcohol. In addition to SD alcohol, aerosol hairsprays also use other VOCs as propellants. The primary purpose of the propellant is to provide pressure to the gas phase in the can, so that the product can be dispensed simply by pressing the valve. The most common propellant currently used in aerosol hairsprays are propane, isobutane, N-butane, dimethylether, HFC 152a, carbon dioxide, nitrous oxide, nitrogen and compressed air.

Chlorofluorocarbons (**KLORO**-floro-kar-bunz) (CFCs) are volatile organic compounds (VOCs) that contain chlorine and were once widely used as propellants in aerosol hairsprays. CFCs have been banned from use in the United States, since 1978, because they destroy the protective ozone in the atmosphere. A single chlorine atom can destroy thousands of ozone molecules.

Although many people still believe that aerosol hairsprays destroy ozone and are more damaging to the environment than pump hairsprays, that is simply not the case. Aerosol hairsprays no longer use CFCs and have the same VOC limits as pump hairsprays.

There is however a real concern about breathing any hairspray, pump or aerosol. And since aerosol hairsprays produce a finer mist, the spray remains in the air longer, which could increase inhalation. You should be cautious and minimize your exposure when using any hairspray. But regardless of which hairspray you use since you will undoubtedly inhale some of it, make sure you use water-soluble hairspray. You can test the solubility of your favorite hairspray very easily. Spray any clean, dry, glass surface with hairspray. Then wait at least 24 hours and try to remove it from the glass. If the hairspray can't be easily removed with warm, soapy water there is a danger it will build up in your lungs.

CONCLUSIONS

Chemical companies are continually researching new surfactants and conditioning agents. They are always looking for improved additives or ingredients. Hair and skin care manufactures are quick to take advantage of new discoveries. Future research should bring many exciting advances.

Unfortunately, it is difficult for hairstylists to distinguish between real, scientific advances and superficial marketing hype. The best way to determine whether a product lives up to its claims is to test it yourself. Don't be afraid to experiment with new ideas or techniques. Testing products will help you find the best ones for your clients, but testing also has another important advantage. Trying new products encourages all manufacturers to improve existing products.

Don't automatically assume that the product will work as advertised. Be honest when evaluating professional products and tools. If your expectations are not met, contact the distributor and ask for advice. If a new technique is involved, it is usually helpful to attend an educational class. Faulty results often lie in improper use or application techniques. Failing to read and/or follow instructions is also a major reason for poor product performance.

REVIEW QUESTIONS

1. What are soaps and how do they differ from shampoo surfactants?

2. Why do surfactant molecules prefer to concentrate in the water/oil interface?

3. How can better wetting of the hair shaft improve salon chemical services?

4. Make a table listing the four major types of surfactants and describe each of their advantages and disadvantages.

5. What is the difference between a humectant and a moisturizer?

6. Why are surfactants superior to soaps?

7. Surfactant is short for _____.

8. Why is it difficult for conditioning chemicals to penetrate deep into the hair shaft? Which types of hair allow the best penetration?

9. Which type of surfactant is also used for conditioning the hair?

DISCUSSION QUESTIONS

1. Why are people so willing to believe, without proof, in folklore ingredients? Until recently, botanicals and herbs were rarely used in shampoos or conditioners. What has changed in our thinking, to create the sudden interest in these types of ingredients?

2. Many hairstylists believe that any ingredient that "coats" the hair shaft cannot be good, because it will weigh down the hair. In this chapter, several important and positive advantages for coating the hair were discussed. Name them and tell why they are important.

3. List all the ways the class can think of to evaluate a new shampoo and conditioner. Would your ideas help you decide whether the new products were better than what you were currently using?

Chapter 11

Color and Hair Lightening

Key Terms

Alkanolamines
Ammonia
Complementary colors
Eumelanin
Frequency
Hydrogen peroxide
Level of color
Melanin
Persulfate salt
Primary colors
Phaeomelanin
Secondary colors
Tone or hue of color
Visible light
Volume
Wavelength

Learning Objectives

After completing this chapter, you should be able to:

- List the factors which influence natural hair color.

- Understand how and why melanin becomes decolorized.

- Describe the role oxidizers play in changing hair color.

- Explain the chemistry of hair lightening.

- Identify the hazards of hair bleaches.

- Recognize porosity gradients and their importance to the colorists.

- Identify ways to work safely with decolorizing chemicals.

We live in a world of color. It influences and shapes our lives in ways we cannot imagine. It is of little wonder that color plays such an important role in the salon.

Exploring the history of hair coloring is like taking a trip through time. Women and men have altered their hair color for thousands of years. Coloring chemicals and tools were discovered in the tombs of pharaohs.

The first synthetic dyes were used to color human hair in 1883. Since that time, science has improved greatly upon the hair coloring process.

Without question, hair coloring products are the most sophisticated and chemically complex salon products available. Developing hair coloring products is a difficult and highly specialized field.

The same holds true for the haircolorist. Becoming a successful color technician takes dedication and skill. The road to this challenge begins here. An understanding of basic color chemistry and theory is an important first step.

VISIBLE LIGHT

What is light? Even though we can see light it doesn't occupy space or have mass, so, it isn't matter. Visible light is energy. The visible light we see with our eyes is actually waves of electromagnetic radiation. Electromagnetic radiation is also called radiant energy because it carries (radiates) energy through space on waves. Radio waves, microwaves, infrared heat, and X-rays are also electromagnetic radiation but are invisible because their wavelengths are beyond the visible spectrum of light.

The wavelength is the only difference between visible light and all other types of electromagnetic radiation. **Visible light** is a small portion of the electromagnetic spectrum with wavelengths between 390 to 760 nm (Figure 11–1). Violet has the shortest wavelength and red has the longest. The wavelength of infrared is just below red, and the wavelength of ultraviolet is just above violet. Infrared and ultraviolet "light" are not really light at all. They are the rays of electromagnetic radiation with wavelengths that are just beyond the visible spectrum.

Waves of electromagnetic radiation are similar to the waves generated when a stone is dropped on the surface of the water. The distance between two successive peaks is the **wavelength** (Figure 11–2). The wavelengths of gamma rays are as small as atomic nuclei, but those of radio waves can be longer than a football field.

Longer wavelengths have lower frequencies (Figure 11–2). They penetrate deeper and are not as energetic as shorter wavelengths. Infrared rays, microwaves, and radio waves have longer wavelengths that are below the visible spectrum.

Shorter wavelengths have higher frequencies (Figure 11–2). They do not penetrate as deeply but are more energetic than longer wavelengths. Ultraviolet rays, X-rays, and gamma rays have shorter wavelengths that are above the visible spectrum.

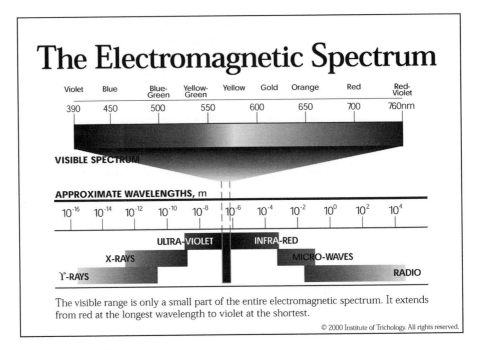

Figure 11-1 *Electromagnetic spectrum.*
(Reprinted with permission of Tri, Institute of Trichology)

Color

The human eye can actually see only a small part of the energy that surrounds us. The eye sees only six basic colors. The multitude of colors we see is the brain's way of visualizing combinations of different wavelengths of the three primary and three secondary colors.

Visible energy is seen as: red, orange, yellow, green, blue, and violet (in order of longest to shortest wavelength)—all the colors of the rainbow. Other energy is invisible (e.g., microwaves, infrared, ultraviolet).

An apple looks red because we see the reflection of red light off its surface. All other wavelengths of color are being absorbed. Our eyes see only the reflected light.

The Laws of Color

The laws of color regulate the mixing of dyes and pigment to make other colors. They are based in science and adapted to art. The laws of color serve as guidelines for harmonious color mixing.

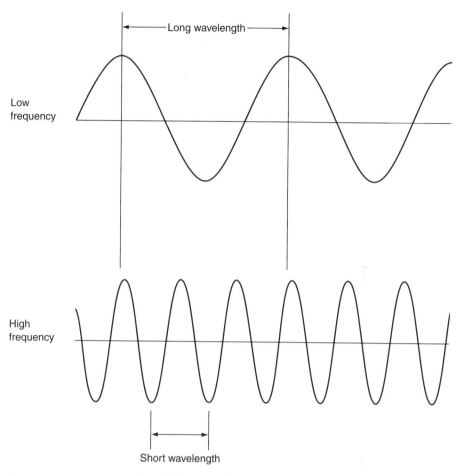

Figure 11-2 *Long wavelengths have low frequency because the number of waves is less frequent (fewer waves) within a given length. Short wavelengths have high frequency because the number of waves is more frequent (more waves) within a given length.*

Primary Colors

Primary colors are basic colors that cannot be created by combining other colors. The three primary colors are yellow, red, and blue. All other colors are created by some combination of yellow, red, or blue.

Secondary Colors

Secondary colors are created by mixing equal amounts of any two primary colors. Mixed in equal parts, yellow and blue create green, blue and red create violet, and red and yellow create orange.

Tertiary Colors

Tertiary colors are created by mixing equal amounts of one primary color with one of its adjacent secondary colors. The tertiary colors are red-violet, blue-violet, blue-green, yellow-green, yellow-orange, and red-orange.

Quarternary Colors

Quarternary colors are all other combinations of all three primary colors.

Complementary Colors

Complementary colors are two colors situated directly across from each other on the color wheel. When mixed together they neutralize each other. For example, when mixed in equal amounts, red and green neutralize each other, creating brown. Orange and blue neutralize each other, and yellow and violet neutralize each other. Complementary colors are always composed of a primary and a secondary color. Complementary pairs always consist of all three primary colors. For example, if you look at the color wheel, you see that the complement of red (a primary color) is green (a secondary color). Green is made up of blue and yellow

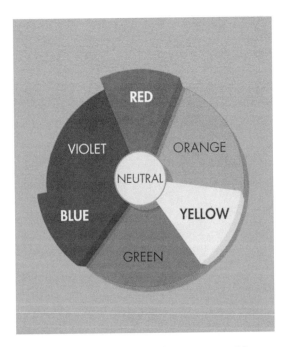

Figure 11-3 *Secondary colors are created from equal parts of any two primaries.*

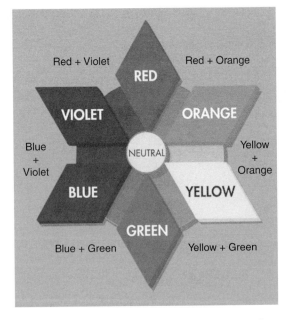

Figure 11-4 *The combination of primary and secondary colors creates tertiary colors.*

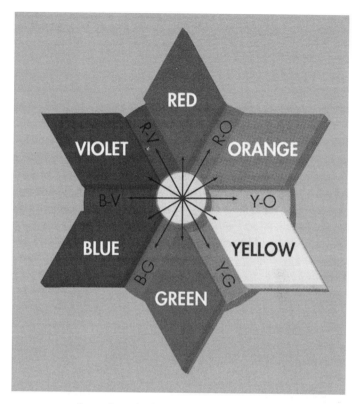

Figure 11–5 *Complete color wheel with arrows to indicate that opposite colors on the color wheel neutralize each other.*

(both primary colors). So, all three primaries are represented in this complementary pair.

Color has two separate components. They are the level of color and the tone or hue of color.

Level of Color

The **level of color** is the saturation, density, or concentration of color. The level of color answers the question, how much color? The level of color is the lightness or darkness of a color. Equal proportions of all three primary colors (red, yellow, and blue) result in white, black, or gray, depending on the concentration. White, black, and gray are all the same color, but they are different levels of the same color. As long as the color has equal parts of all three primary colors, the resulting color will be white, black, or gray depending on the concentration.

A number value from 1 to 10 is usually used to express the level of color. Black is a level 1. Black is the darkest possible color with the highest concentration of pigment. White is a level 10, the lightest possible color with the least

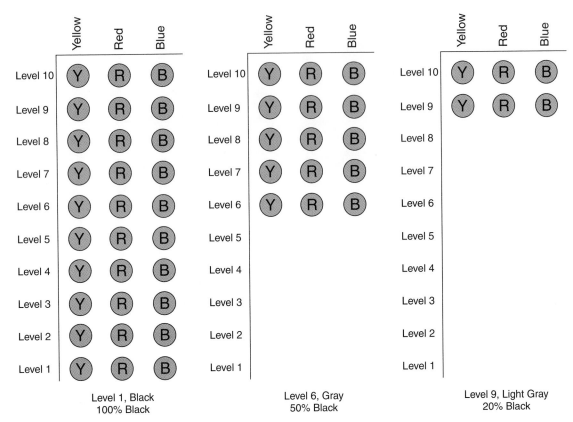

Figure 11-6 *Equal parts of all three primary colors make white, black or gray, depending on the concentration. Ten parts of black without any white makes the color a level 1 black.*

Figure 11-7 *Five parts of black and five parts of white make a level 6 gray.*

Figure 11-8 *Two parts of black and eight parts of white make a level 9, light gray.*

concentration of pigment. Levels 2 through 9 are all different shades of gray, depending on the concentration (Figs. 11–6 to 11–8).

Tone or Hue of Color

The **tone** or **hue of color** is the balance of the colors. The tone or hue answers the question, which colors? Unequal proportions of all three primary colors (yellow, red, and blue) result in browns or blonds, depending on the concentration or level of color. A natural brown or blond hair color is composed of three parts yellow, two parts red, and one part blue (Figs. 11–9 and 11–10). The hair will be brown or blond depending on the concentration of color, but all natural colors have the same balance.

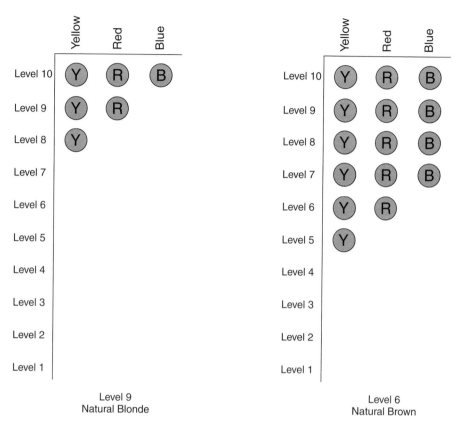

Figure 11-9 A typical beige blond or natural brown is made from three parts of yellow, two parts of red and one part of blue.

Figure 11-10 A level 6, natural brown.

A name is usually given to express the tone or hue of color. Some examples are strawberry blond, chestnut brown, and flame red. Many haircolor companies use letters to indicate the tone of color. Some examples are G for gold, R for red, OR for orange red, or RV for red-violet.

Melanin (MEL-uh-nin) is the pigment responsible for natural hair color. The wide range of hair colors comes from the two types of melanin found in cortex, eumelanin and phaeomelanin. White hair contains neither type of melanin. White is the color of keratin without the influence of melanin.

Eumelanin is the most common type and gives hair shades from brown to black.

Phaeomelanin gives hair yellowish-blond tones and ginger and red colors.

Three factors determine all natural hair colors from light blond to jet black:

1. The thickness of the hair

2. The total number and size of pigment granules

3. The ratio of eumelanin to phaeomelanin

LIGHTENING THE HAIR

Hair is bleached or lightened by decolorizing the melanin. Decolorizing does not remove the melanin. The chemical structure of melanin is altered so that it no longer absorbs visible light. Decolorizing the hair makes it reflect instead of absorb light. If the hair reflects all the light from a white light source, we see the hair as white. To lighten dark hair to white is difficult and extremely damaging. Dark hair is rarely lightened beyond the pale yellow stage.

Natural-looking hair colors are composed of three parts yellow, two parts red, and one part blue. The concentration of color determines the level. The darkest natural brown and the lightest natural blond have the same balance of color; only the concentration is different (Figures 11–9 and 11–10).

Decolorizing natural hair color doesn't just make it lighter; it also changes the balance or tone of the color, which makes it warmer. Remember that the three primary colors are yellow, red, and blue, and all natural-looking hair colors are composed of three parts yellow, two parts red, and one part blue. Lightening hair removes all three primary colors in equal proportions. Subtracting one part of each of the three primary colors from a natural color leaves two parts yellow and one part red, which is orange (Figure 11–18).

The results of decolorizing natural pigment will vary depending on the original underlying color. Light hair colors will usually lighten quickly and easily. Darker hair is often much more difficult and may not lighten beyond a yellow-gold stage. This unwanted brassy tone can be neutralized with a toner. Depositing a blue toner will neutralize orange hair (Figure 11–19). Note that depositing a blue toner in pale yellow hair will cause the hair to turn green. (Figures 11–20 and 11–21).

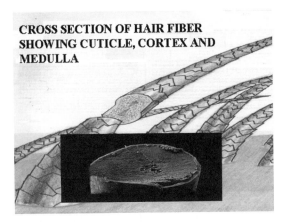

CROSS SECTION OF HAIR FIBER SHOWING CUTICLE, CORTEX AND MEDULLA

Figure 11-11 *Cross section of hair fiber showing cuticle, cortex ,and medulla.*
(Reprinted with permisson of Clairol, Inc.)

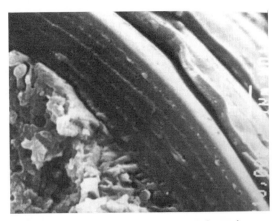

Figure 11-12 *High magnification of cuticle scales overlapping the cortex. Note the melanin pigment shown as dark spots.*
(Reprinted with permission of Clairol Inc.)

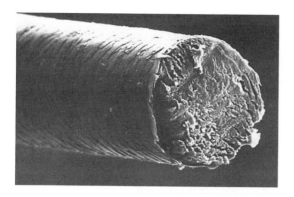

Figure 11-13 *Cross section of hair showing exposed cortex.*
(Reprinted with permission of Clairol, Inc.)

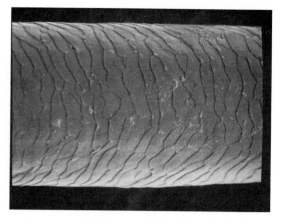

Figure 11-14 *Hair strand with closed cuticle.*
(Reprinted with permission of Clairol, Inc.)

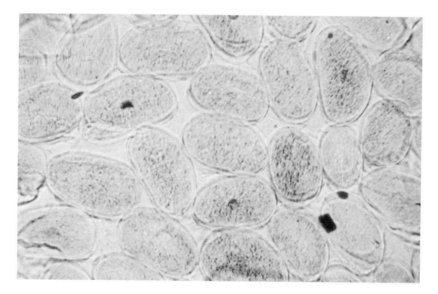

Figure 11-15 *Cross section of hairs showing natural pigments in auburn hair.* (Note *the absence of color in cuticle.)*
(Courtesy: C. V. Stead, I.C.A. and American Perfumer)

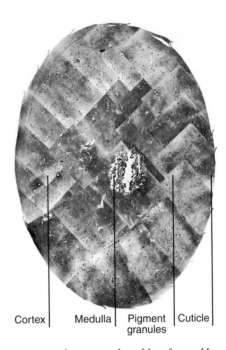

Cortex | Medulla | Pigment granules | Cuticle

Figure 11-16 A cross section of an entire hair fiber, formed by taking a series of photos that were assembled to create a composite picture, magnified 1,400 times. Note especially the layers of the cuticle, the cortex, and the medulla. Of special interest are the thousands of pigment (color) granules which are so important in hair lightening. (*Courtesy: Gillette Company Research Institute, Rockville, Maryland*)

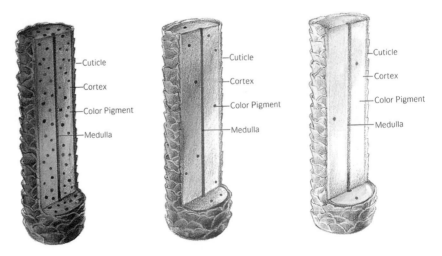

Figure 11-17 Hair lighteners decolorize melanin in the cortex.

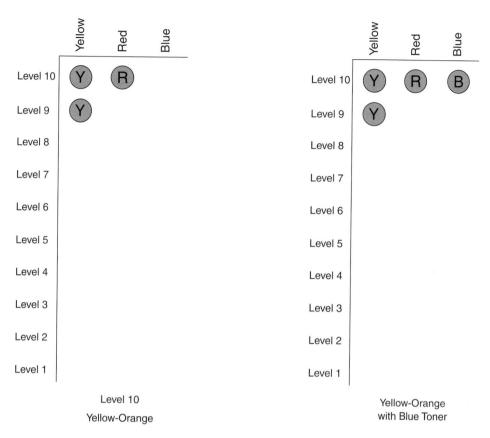

Figure 11-18 *Hair lightened to an unwanted, brassy, level 10, yellow-orange.*

Figure 11-19 *Adding a blue toner to level 10, yellow-orange corrects unwanted brassy tone.*

Ten Degrees or Stages of Decolorization

There are ten degrees of decolorization or stages that are involved in hair lightening from a level 1 to a level 10. Each natural hair color starts the decolorization process at a different stage. Only black hair will pass through all ten stages.

Level 10	Pale Yellow
Level 9	Yellow
Level 8	Yellow-Gold
Level 7	Gold
Level 6	Orange-Gold
Level 5	Orange
Level 4	Red-Orange

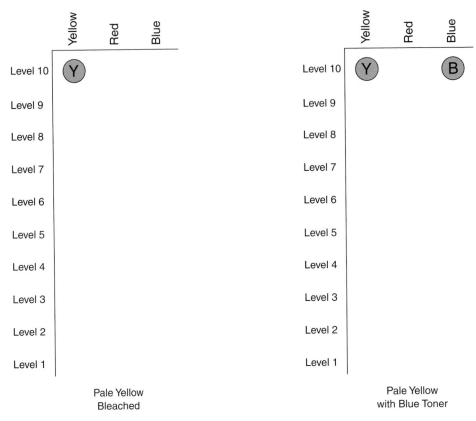

Figure 11-20 *Hair lightened to a level 10, pale yellow.*

Figure 11-21 *Adding a blue toner to level 10, pale yellow results in green hair.*

Level 3   Red

Level 2   Red-Brown

Level 1   Dark Red-Brown

Lighteners are used for two purposes:

1. As a color treatment, to lighten hair to its final shade.

2. To prepare the hair for the application of toners.

The sun's ultraviolet rays are powerful enough to decolorize melanin, but the process is a gradual one and difficult to control. Natural-looking highlights are often referred to as sun streaks but are rarely achieved naturally. Modern salon highlighting methods consistently produce natural-looking results with a minimum of damage. Hair lightening is achieved by oxidation of melanin within the cortex of the hair.

Oxidation Reactions

Since hydrogen peroxide causes oxidation reactions, it is called an oxidizer. The first recorded use of hydrogen peroxide as a hair bleach was in 1860. It was used by the mistress of Napoleon III, presumably to please his majesty.

The chemical symbol for **hydrogen peroxide** is H_2O_2. Hydrogen peroxide can be thought of as water (H_2O) with an extra atom of oxygen. This reactive extra oxygen atom is responsible for hydrogen peroxide's ability to oxidize melanin into colorless compounds. This oxidation reaction is responsible for the decolorization of melanin in the hair.

Pure hydrogen peroxide is far too strong to be used in salons. Hairstylists use a solution of hydrogen peroxide diluted with water. The term **volume** indicates the percentage of hydrogen peroxide in the solution. Twenty volume hydrogen peroxide is a solution of 6 percent hydrogen peroxide and 94 percent water. Different volumes of hydrogen peroxide indicate different concentrations. Higher volumes are more concentrated solutions. Lower volumes are less concentrated solutions (Figs. 11–22 and 11–23).

Note that one ounce of 40 volume peroxide contains the same amount of peroxide as two ounces of 20 volume. The only difference between the two is the amount of water. The 20 volume peroxide is simply less concentrated (Fig. 11–24).

Since hydrogen peroxide is composed of water and oxygen gas, it shouldn't be surprising that the decomposition of hydrogen peroxide yields oxygen gas and water. The term *volume* refers to the volume of oxygen gas that is released when hydrogen peroxide decomposes. Decomposition of one ounce of 20 volume peroxide yields twenty ounces of oxygen gas and one ounce of water. Decomposition of one ounce of 10 volume peroxide yields ten ounces of oxygen gas and one ounce of water.

Cream developers are emulsions of hydrogen peroxide, water, and creaming agents. A variety of creaming agents can be added including fatty alcohols, alkanolamides, and ethoxylated alkyl phenols. These materials thicken the developer and make it opaque. They also contribute to the thickness of the formulation after mixing. Some even act as conditioners.

Solutions of hydrogen peroxide are acid-stabilized to prevent premature breakdown. Hydrogen peroxide is unstable. Light, dirt, oils, or other contaminants cause rapid decomposition to oxygen and water. Metal utensils and bowls also decompose hydrogen peroxide. Never store hydrogen peroxide in sealed, metal containers. The rapid breakdown creates a high-pressure buildup of oxygen which can cause the container to rupture.

Peroxide should be stored in accordance with manufacturer's instructions. Store hydrogen peroxide in a cool location, in its original container.

To avoid contamination, never pour anything back into the original container. For added safety, always wear gloves when using or mixing hydrogen peroxide.

OXIDIZERS IN USE

Oxidizing agents may be highly corrosive to the eyes, skin, and lungs. Hydrogen peroxide and other oxidizers work by releasing oxygen. Since we breathe oxygen, some mistakenly believe that oxidizers are safe and cannot cause harm. This is not the case. Oxidizers are potentially hazardous and must be used with care.

Although it is possible to work safely with oxidizers, special precautions must be taken. Always wear safety glasses and protective gloves when mixing or using an oxidizer. High-volume peroxides and bromates are especially dangerous to the eyes.

Oxidizers are corrosive and can cause serious burns, scarring, and skin damage. Wear a suitable dust mask when dispensing dry, powdered oxidizers. This prevents inhalation of the corrosive powders.

Carefully read the Material Safety Data Sheet (MSDS) and instructions for all salon products, especially corrosives and oxidizers. Follow the recommended manufacturer's procedure and precautions. This is important for everyone's safety.

STRENGTH OF HYDROGEN PEROXIDE SOLUTIONS	
Percent Hydrogen Peroxide in Water	Peroxide Volume
3%	10 volume
6%	20 volume
9%	30 volume
12%	40 volume
30%	100 volume
35%	130 volume

Note: Extra special care should be taken when handling solutions above 30 volume. Never exceed the manufacturer's recommendations.

Figure 11-22 *Strengths of hydrogen peroxide which compare the volume of peroxide to the concentration of peroxide.*

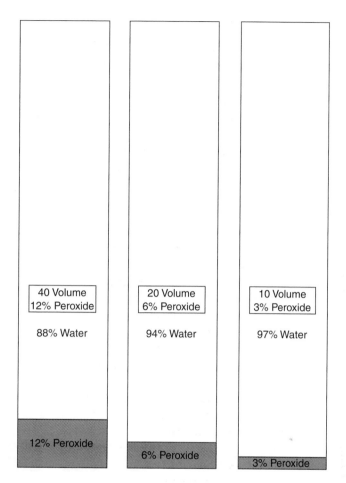

Figure 11-23 *Equal amounts of 10, 20, and 40 volume peroxide, showing the concentration of peroxide and water as a percentages.*

pH and Hair Lightening

Hair lighteners usually have a pH between 9.5 and 10. Effective hair lighteners must have an alkaline pH for two reasons. First, an alkaline pH softens, swells, and opens the cuticle to allow the lightener to penetrate into the cortex. Remember that the melanin is located within the cortex. Solutions with a higher pH swell the hair more, penetrate deeper, and increase the decolorization of the hair.

Second, an alkaline pH triggers the rapid decomposition of hydrogen peroxide and speeds up the decolorization process. Hydrogen peroxide is acid-stabilized to prevent premature decomposition. When used alone, hydrogen

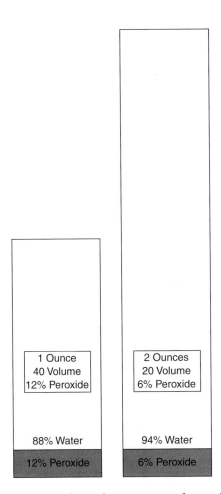

Figure 11-24 *This illustration shows that one ounce of 40 volume peroxide contains the same amount of peroxide as two ounces of 20 volume peroxide. The 40 volume simply contains less water.*

peroxide oxidizes slowly and lightens the hair very little. Mixing hydrogen peroxide with an alkaline hair lightener raises the pH of the hydrogen peroxide and triggers the release of the extra oxygen.

Ammonia

Ammonia (uh-**MOH**-nee-uh) has been safely used as an alkalizing agent in hair lighteners for decades. Ammonia is an inorganic alkali because it does not contain carbon. Ammonia is a small, volatile molecule that evaporates quickly, which accounts for its strong odor. Although ammonia is more effective for hair lightening than other alkalizing agents, its use is declining because of its strong, offensive odor.

The chemical formula for ammonia is NH_3. Ammonia is alkaline and raises the pH by removing a hydrogen ion (H^+) from water, which leaves an alkaline hydroxide ion (OH^-). Remember, from Chapter 9, Advanced Chemistry, that all alkalis derive their chemical reactivity from the hydroxide ion (OH^-).

$$NH_3 + H_2O \rightarrow NH_4{}^+ + \mathbf{OH^-}$$

Alkanolamines

Alkanolamines (al-kan-all-**AM**-eenz) are also used as alkalizing agents in hair lighteners. They are used to replace ammonia and are gaining in popularity because of their low odor. These large, organic molecules contain carbon and are not as volatile as ammonia, so there is little or no odor associated with their use. *Aminomethylpropanol* (AMP) (uh-**MEE**-noh-meth-yl-pro-pan-all), and *monoethanolamine* (MEA) (mahn-oh-**ETH**-an-all-am-een), are examples of common organic alkalis that are used instead of ammonia. Although they eliminate the ammonia odor, they may not be as effective at lightening the hair as ammonia.

Alkanolamines are formed by a chemical reaction of ammonia with ethylene oxide, which gives a mix of MEA, DEA, and TEA. Even though alkanolamines may not smell as strong as ammonia, they can be every bit as alkaline and every bit as damaging to the hair. Many harsh chemicals have little or no odor. Remember that carbon monoxide is an odorless, deadly poison. Contrary to what your nose and the marketing department may tell you, ammonia free does not necessarily mean free of damage.

Alkanolamines raise the pH of a solution in exactly the same way that ammonia does. The chemical formula for monoethanolamine is $HOCH_2CH_2NH_2$. The amino or amine functional group is (NH_2), which acts just like ammonia (NH_3). Remember, from Chapter 9, that all alkalis derive their chemical reactivity from the hydroxide ion (OH^-).

$$HOCH_2CH_2 - NH_2 + H_2O \rightarrow HOCH_2CH_2 - NH_4{}^+ + \mathbf{OH^-}$$

Effects of Bleaching/Lightening on the Hair

Melanin is not the only thing attacked by an alkaline pH and peroxide mixture. Keratin is also susceptible to oxidation. Both the salt bonds (ionic bonds) and disulfide bonds (sulfur bonds) in the cortex are exposed. The extent of damage to these bonds depends on the solution's strength, the pH level, and the length of treatment. Carefully controlling the bleaching process minimizes keratin damage.

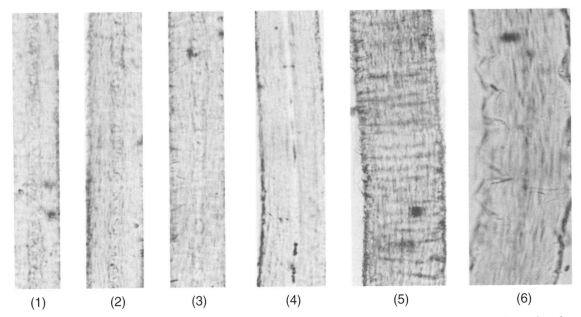

(1)   (2)   (3)   (4)   (5)   (6)

Figure 11-25 *Effects of pH on lightened (bleached) hair. The numbered specimens show the effects of acids and alkalies on the diameter and imbrications of bleached hair. (1. strong acid, pH-3.0; 2. mild acid, pH-5.0; 3. neutral (water), pH-7.0; 4. mild alkali, pH-08.5; 5. strong alkali, pH-9.5; 6. excessive alkali [depilatory action — note twist of hair before dissolving], pH-12.0)*

Never use more than the recommended amount of activator. Extreme damage to the hair and scalp, or even hair loss, may occur. Using higher than recommended volumes or adding "peroxide boosters" is equally hazardous (Fig. 11–25).

Bleached hair no longer behaves like natural hair. The hair becomes more porous, therefore taking longer to dry. It may feel rougher and brittle and may tangle easily. Hair strength can be dramatically lowered. The individual strands stretch easier. The increased porosity lowers resistance to future bleaching and other chemical services. Damaged, porous hair absorbs more dyes and conditioners.

A slight or normal bleach application causes minor changes in the hair structure. The loss of strength and porosity increase is minimal. Proper conditioning and care should restore the hair's appearance and softness. A controlled increase in porosity can be beneficial since tints and toners absorb better after lightening.

Heavy or repeated bleaching drastically alters the hair. A single, extensive bleach application can lower the hair's strength by 15 percent. Multiple treatments can decrease the hair's strength even further as the proteins are frequently stripped from the cortex. The scalp may be left dry and irritated (Figures 11–26 to 11–30).

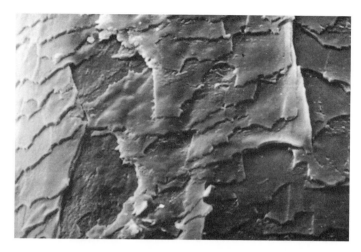

Figure 11-26 *Bleaching causes the cuticle layers to swell, becoming raised and roughened.*
(Courtesy: Redken Laboratories, Inc.)

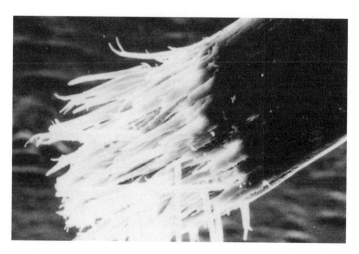

Figure 11-27 *Overlightened hair ends split and fray.*
(Courtesy: Redken Laboratories, Inc.)

Semi-permanent and permanent oxidation dyes are far more difficult to lighten or lift than natural melanin. Only experienced hairstylists should attempt removal of dyes. Strand testing is of great value and can help lessen hair damage. Strand testing gives important information about the reaction of the hair, and should always be performed to ensure high-quality results (Fig. 11–31).

Proper care and attention can help avoid excessive hair and scalp damage.

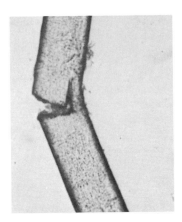

Figure 11-28 *Lightened hair with broken shaft.*
(Courtesy: Gillette Company Research Institute Rockville, Maryland)

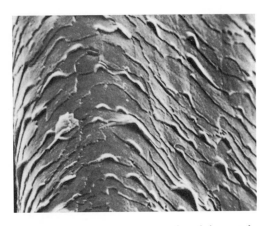

Figure 11-29 *Damage to scales of the cuticle caused by lightening (bleaching) magnified 2,100 times.*
(Courtesy: Gillette Company Research Laboratories, Inc.)

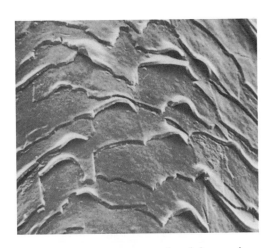

Figure 11-30 *Damage to scales of the cuticle caused by lightening (bleaching) magnified 4,200 times.*
(Courtesy: Gillette Company Research Laboratories, Inc.)

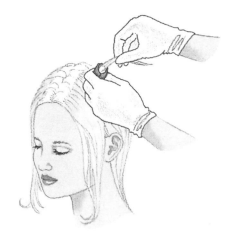

Figure 11-31 *Strand testing.*

Bleaching/Lightening Safety

Bleach often comes in contact with the scalp during application. The high alkalinity and presence of an oxidizer can cause dermatitis. Clients often experience tightness and drying of the scalp. Keeping the bleaching product off the skin eliminates this problem.

The scalp has a protective barrier of sebum that shampoo applications temporarily remove. Ask clients to refrain from shampooing their hair for twenty-four hours before lightening. You may recommend clients use a shampoo to remove spray and styling aid residue before the appointment. Unless absolutely necessary, never shampoo a client's hair before a bleach application.

Carefully examine the scalp and hair before a bleach application. Look for signs of scalp irritation, redness, tender or puffy tissue, open sores, excessive dryness, or other skin problems. If you spot problems, advise the client to see a dermatologist before proceeding with any chemical applications.

Pay attention to the client's hair porosity. Healthy, virgin hair near the scalp and damaged porous ends will cause varying degrees of lightening. *Porosity gradients* refers to a noticeable increase in porosity from the scalp to the hair ends. The porous keratin is affected more quickly by bleach applications. This difference may result in extensive damage if not treated carefully. The mid-strand is more resistant and requires a longer bleaching time. Timing and porosity questions can be answered by performing a strand test.

There are other important considerations besides porosity. Generally, hair near the scalp is affected more rapidly by any chemical treatment. Remember this when applying lightening products. Heat from the scalp and head speeds the chemical reaction. A good rule to remember is, "The rate of a chemical reaction is doubled if the temperature is raised by 18°F/10°C."

Performing a recommended strand test is important for many reasons. Strand tests help you identify procedures to avoid serious errors caused by variables such as porosity gradients, temperature changes, and improper mixing or application.

A common mistake is made when touching up re-growth, if care is not taken to avoid overlapping. Overlapping the bleach onto previously lightened hair will result in breakage and excessive damage (Fig. 11–32).

The lightening process is completed with proper shampooing and rinsing. Alkaline residues are trapped in the keratin if the hair is not properly shampooed and rinsed. Failing to properly neutralize the residues will cause continuing damage. To neutralize residues completely, rinse the hair with an acid rinse, shampoo with a mild, acid shampoo, and apply a conditioner. Take care to massage the scalp gently to prevent further irritation to sensitive scalp tissue.

Types of Bleaching Products

Hair lighteners come in many forms (i.e., pastes, creams, oils, shampoos, gels, and powders). Each type uses oxidizers, but they have some important differences.

Creams are easy to use and run less. They are prepared by adding thickeners to alkaline substances. Fatty material conditioning agents are included to help minimize damage. Alkaline cream is then used to thicken and activate hydrogen peroxide. Thickened products also have the advantage of controlling ammonia loss through evaporation.

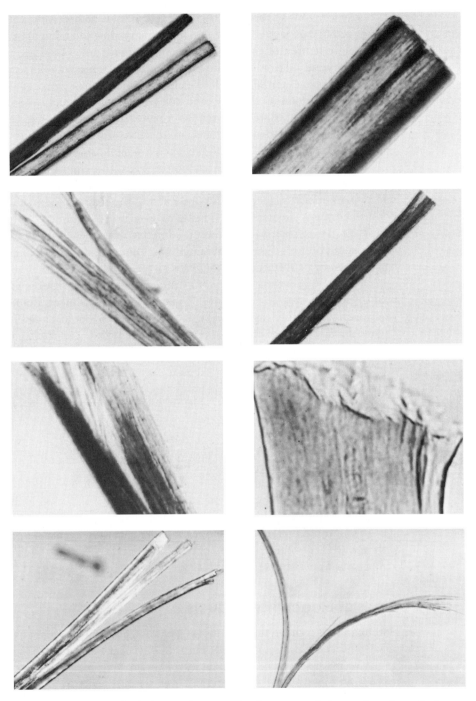

Figure 11-32 Illustrations of split hair ends caused by the misuse of chemical products (lighteners, tints, or permanent-wave solutions) in the performance of hair services.

Sometimes a *bleaching powder* is added instead of hydrogen peroxide. These powders are different chemical forms of peroxide and must be handled with care. Follow each of the safe-handling precautions suggested for peroxide and oxidizers. Use a dust mask when mixing and measuring to avoid inhaling the corrosive powders.

Blue or violet dyes are often added to bleaches to offset yellow tones.

Oil or gel bleaching products have several important advantages. First, they are transparent and allow the user to follow the progress of the lightener more easily than opaque products. Second, oils prevent the scalp from becoming too dry.

Follow each of these product applications with an acid rinse and a mild, acid shampoo.

Powdered Off-the-Scalp Hair Lighteners

Hair lightening is done at an alkaline pH with a high concentration of hydrogen peroxide. But the degree of lightening obtained in this process is limited, regardless of the pH or the concentration of hydrogen peroxide.

In order to overcome this limitation, a **persulfate salt** is usually added to powdered off-the-scalp hair lighteners. Ammonium persulfate, sodium persulfate and/or potassium persulfate are usually used. These ingredients are only used in powdered lighteners because they must be packaged in a powdered form. Powdered off-the-scalp hair lighteners are only recommended for off-the-scalp applications because although the addition of persulfate salts increases lightening ability, it also increases scalp irritation.

Powdered, off-the-scalp hair lighteners are a mixture of several different ingredients, which will often separate during storage and shipping. Failure to thoroughly mix the powder, prior to use, can result in a non-uniform mixture of these ingredients. If the powder is not thoroughly mixed prior to use, the ingredients on the top may not be the same ingredients that are on the bottom. Improper mixing can cause erratic results or extreme damage to the hair. Excessive heat may develop, which can put the client in danger.

PERSONAL SAFETY

Remember the rules for working safely. They are especially important when working with powerful oxidizers. If care is not taken or if the manufacturer's instruction is ignored, serious injury can result. If oxidizers can cause dermatitis to the scalp, they can easily and quickly damage the skin or eyes. However, if you take the time to master the products and application techniques you should have few problems.

REVIEW QUESTIONS

1. Why does red look different from blue?
2. What factors are responsible for natural hair color?
3. How do oxidizers lighten the color of hair?
4. List all of the potential hazards associated with oxidizers.
5. What safety equipment should be used whenever working with oxidizers?
6. Give two reasons why an alkalizing agent is added to hydrogen peroxide.
7. Which is the stronger peroxide solution, 6 percent or 30 volume?
8. Why should hydrogen peroxide never be placed in a dusty container?
9. Why is hydrogen peroxide sold in dark, plastic containers?
10. List all of the effects of overbleaching.

DISCUSSION QUESTIONS

1. When lightening new hair growth, is it acceptable to overlap previously bleached hair?
2. Why is strand testing important? Is it really worth the time and effort if you are an expert at lightening hair?

Chapter 12

Haircoloring

Key Terms

Compound dyes
Fillers
Long-lasting semi-permanent
   or demi-permanent colors
Metallic dyes
Nonoxidation colors
Oxidation colors
Permanent colors
Temporary colors
Toners
Traditional semi-permanent
   colors

Learning Objectives

After completing this chapter, you should be able to:

- List the basic types of haircoloring products.

- Explain the chemistry of haircoloring.

- List the various types and function of ingredients found in hair colors.

- Understand the concept of color lightening, filling, and toning.

- Describe techniques for safe color removal.

- Recognize and avoid the danger presented by metallic home coloring.

- Avoid the potential risks associated with coloring chemicals.

INTRODUCTION

The demand for professional haircoloring services has increased dramatically over the last few years. In many salons, haircoloring now accounts for 50 percent of a salon's total service sales. The increased demand for haircoloring services has resulted in a dramatic increase in the number and type of new haircoloring products that are available for salon use.

Today's hair color technicians find themselves armed with impressive, sophisticated tools. As products and application techniques advance, the demand grows for professional color technicians. The demands placed on color technicians continue to grow, as well.

Learn the how and why of hair coloring and you will be ready for any new technology.

HAIR COLOR THEORY

A detailed, step-by-step, guide to proper color application techniques can be found in *Milady's Standard Textbook of Cosmetology*. This chapter focuses on the theory behind hair coloring techniques.

TYPES OF HAIRCOLORING PRODUCTS

There are two main categories of professional haircoloring products marketed for salon use and two different types of products in each category. Appendix E contains Material Safety Data Sheets (MSDS) that show the ingredients for different haircoloring products.

1. Nonoxidation Colors

   a. Temporary

   b. Traditional semi-permanent

2. Oxidation colors

   a. Long lasting semi-permanent or demi-permanent

   b. Permanent

Nonoxidation Colors

Nonoxidation colors contain only one component. They are used directly as they come out of the bottle and are not mixed with developer or activator. There is no chemical reaction involved and no new chemicals are formed. The change in the hair is only physical. Nonoxidation colors deposit stable, direct dyes that have been formed prior to the application of the color. The color in the bottle is the color deposited on the hair. Nonoxidation colors can only deposit color and are not able to lighten natural hair color. Nonoxidation colors create a physical change in the hair and will shampoo out without leaving a noticeable regrowth. There are two types of nonoxidation haircolors: temporary and traditional semi-permanent.

Temporary Colors

Temporary colors are cosmetics in the truest sense. Coloring occurs on the hair's surface, without chemically altering keratin. The hair is coated with a color which absorbs and reflects light differently from natural melanin.

There are both advantages and disadvantages to temporary haircoloring products. Temporary color products are a color mask. They cover the natural melanin and reflect different wavelengths of light to the eyes. Temporary color products cannot make the hair lighter than the original color. Since the keratin is unaltered, washing off the color coating returns the hair to its original color.

The disadvantages are also considered the two major advantages of these products. Temporary color products are quickly removed by shampooing and no chemical changes are made to the keratin. These products are safe and easy to use. However, applying dark coloring to light blond hair should be done carefully. The darker colors may cause staining, especially on porous hair. Temporary coloring molecules are far too large to pass through the cuticles of healthy hair. However, highly porous hair may allow some color to penetrate.

Temporary colorings come in a variety of forms, ranging from concentrated water-based solutions, shampoos, and colored conditioners to setting lotions, foams, and sprays.

Colored settings lotions and foams are the most interesting. These products take advantage of new technology. Softened polymer films are dissolved in a solvent and mixed with the hair coloring. Upon drying, a think transparent polymer film coats the hair shaft with coloring. Polymer film products have a few benefits over the other types. The films prevent color penetration, even on porous hair. The higher viscosity (thickness) improves control during application (Figure 12–1).

Traditional Semi-Permanent Colors (Direct Dyes)

Traditional semi-permanent colors should resist at least four shampooings. Better coloring results are obtained if the hair is slightly porous.

Traditional semi-permanent colors are also called direct colors because they do not need to develop color. They are similar to temporary colors. The important difference is the coloring product's affinity (a-**FIN**-i-tee) for keratin. Affinity describes how tightly the color molecule bonds to keratin. Greater affinity means longer-lasting color. By using small color molecules, solvents, alkaline swelling agents, and surfactants, a greater amount of color enters the cortex. However, most of the color absorbs into the outer layer staining the cuticle.

Sometimes, color mixtures selectively color the hair. For example, chestnut brown shades are made by blending a red-orange color with a malachite green

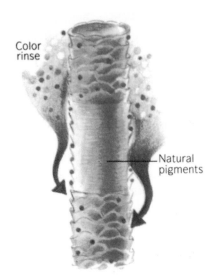

Color rinse

Natural pigments

Figure 12-1 *Action of temporary hair color.*

color. Porous, damaged ends may absorb large amounts of green and less red-orange. The results would be green-colored-tipped hair.

Better color permanence is achieved if the coloring enters and stains the cortex. Alkaline materials are used to raise the pH level. The increased pH value lifts the cuticle slightly and allows better penetration.

Some colors are designed to link with the salt bonds in the cortex. This greatly increases color affinity. Semi-permanent colors are sometimes used to brighten permanently colored hair.

The mild alkalinity of semi-permanent colors creates little damage to the hair. However, as with most alkaline products, after the service the hair should be shampooed with a mild, acid shampoo and followed by an acid conditioner or rinse. This neutralizes alkaline residues and restores hair to normal pH levels (Figure 12–2).

Oxidation Colors

Oxidation colors contain two components. They are not used directly as they come out of the bottle. Oxidation colors must be mixed with developer or activator immediately before use. The oxidizing agent in the developer causes an oxidation reaction that develops the color. The dyes in oxidation colors are unstable until they are developed and are deposited in the hair as they are formed. The color in the original bottle is not the color deposited on the hair. The final color

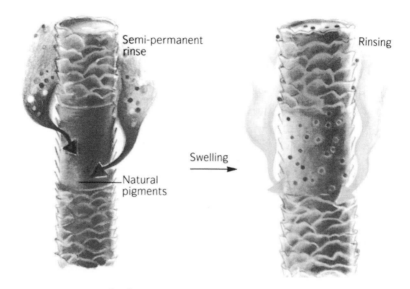

Figure12-2 *Increased color penetration with semi-permanent dyes.*

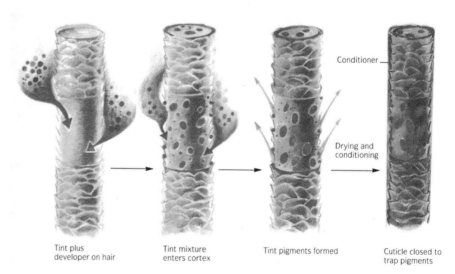

| Tint plus developer on hair | Tint mixture enters cortex | Tint pigments formed | Cuticle closed to trap pigments |

Figure12-3 *Action of permanent hair color.*

is developed, on the hair, during processing. Permanent oxidation colors can deposit color and lighten natural hair color in one application. Oxidation colors create a chemical change in the hair and will not shampoo out as quickly as nonoxidation colors.

FORMULATION AND CHEMISTRY

Oxidation colors are chemically complex but easy to use. The active ingredients can be mixed in many forms (i.e., creams, emulsions, gels, and shampoos).

Primary intermediates are the major color-producing chemicals. Upon oxidation primary intermediates create various colors. Oxidation colors rarely contain less than two primary intermediates and some may have four or more.

Modifiers or couplers are included to create complex color blends. Secondary and tertiary colors require four to six modifiers. Modifiers chemically combine with the primary intermediates. This process is similar to building a tiny ship in a bottle. Once constructed, the ship cannot be removed. The same holds true for the final dye molecule. It is too big to escape through the cuticle.

Modifiers and primary intermediates chemically construct the final dye molecule inside the cortex.

Several direct colors are added to help adjust the hair's highlights. Then the solution is made alkaline. Finally, antioxidant stabilizers are blended into the mixture/formula to prevent premature oxidation. These additives prevent the final dye molecules from being constructed until the color is activated with hydrogen peroxide. Antioxidants also slow down the oxidizer (peroxide), allowing more time for tint application.

The chemical reactions that create the dye molecule are extremely complex. Scientists still do not completely understand them. Before producing the final color, these chemical cocktails undergo dozens of different chemical reactions.

There are two types of oxidation haircolors: long-lasting semi-permanent or demi-permanent colors, and permanent colors.

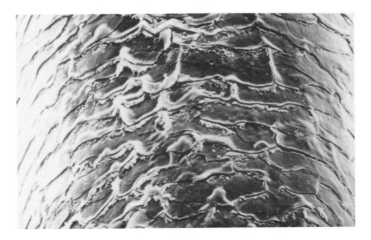

Figure12-4 *High-lift tint damage.*

(Courtesy: Redken Laboratories, Inc.)

Long-Lasting Semi-Permanent or Demi-Permanent Colors (No Lift-Deposit Only)

Long-lasting semi-permanent or demi-permanent colors deposit long-lasting color, without lightening the natural hair color. They are often called no lift-deposit only colors. They can be used for covering gray hair or enhancing the color of pigmented hair. Long-lasting semi-permanent colors usually last from four to six weeks. Since they do not lighten the natural hair color, they are considered semi-permanent.

Long-lasting semi-permanent oxidation colors are usually milder than permanent oxidation colors. They are able to deposit without lifting because they are usually less alkaline than permanent colors and are mixed with a low volume developer. You should remember, from pH and hair lightening in Chapter 11, that hair decolorization requires a high pH and a high concentration of peroxide.

Many long-lasting semi-permanent and demi-permanent colors use alkalizing agents other than ammonia and oxidizing agents other than hydrogen peroxide. It's important to note that these products are not necessarily any less damaging because of the type of alkalizing agent or oxidizer that is used. If they are milder, it's because the concentration of these active ingredients is less.

Permanent Colors (Lift and Deposit)

Besides creating beautiful, long-lasting color, permanent oxidation colors offer other advantages. **Permanent colors** can lighten and deposit color at the same time, and in one process. They are able to lighten natural hair color because they are more alkaline than long-lasting semi-permanent oxidation colors and are usually mixed with a higher volume developer.

The amount of lift is controlled by the pH of the color and the concentration of peroxide in the developer. The amount of lift increases as the pH of the color and the concentration of peroxide increases. Most permanent colors are mixed with peroxide in equal parts, or a 1:1 ratio. Permanent haircolors are usually mixed with equal parts of 20 volume peroxide and lift one or two levels. Permanent colors mixed with equal parts of 30 volume peroxide lift about three levels and when mixed with equal parts of 40 volume peroxide, permanent colors lift up to four levels.

Changing the ratio of peroxide to haircolor also changes the final concentration of peroxide in the finished color mixture. Some permanent oxidative colors recommend mixing two parts of 20 volume peroxide with one part haircolor (double peroxide). This increases the ratio of peroxide to color from 1:1, to 2:1 and increases the final concentration of peroxide in the finished color mixture by 25 percent. Mixing 20 volume peroxide with haircolor in a 2:1 ratio increases the effective volume of peroxide in the finished color mixture from 20 volume to 27 volume.

Some ultra-high lift permanent oxidative colors recommend mixing a double amount of 40 volume peroxide, which increases the volume of peroxide in the

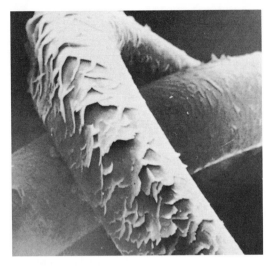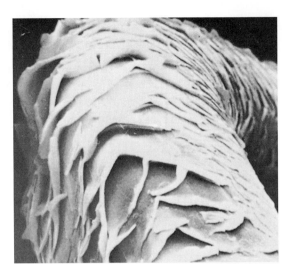

Figure 12–5 *Lightened hair tied into a knot, shown magnified 630 times (left) and 2,100 times (right), emphasizes the cuticle damage caused by lightening.*
(Courtesy: Gillette Company Research Institute, Rockville, Maryland)

finished color mixture from 40 volume to 54 volume. Although ultra-high lift permanent colors deposit as they lighten hair, they can create just as much damage as any other on the scalp hairlightener. There is no way to lighten hair without damaging it. The amount of damage to the hair increases as the lift of the color increases.

Permanent oxidation colors don't always lighten the natural color even though they have that ability. For a deposit only effect with no lifting of the natural hair color, some permanent oxidation colors recommend mixing equal parts of 5 volume or 10 volume peroxide. These are the same low concentrations of peroxide used in semi-permanent long-lasting colors. These low concentrations of peroxide are sufficient to develop the dye in the color, but unable to create any noticeable lightening of the natural color, even at a slightly higher pH.

Never exceed the manufacturer's recommended peroxide volume. Additional alkaline material should never be added to speed up processing. Violating the fundamental rules of cosmetology can cause serious damage to a client's hair and scalp.

Color Fillers

A slight degree of porosity can enhance tint absorption. Porosity gradients, however, may cause uneven lightening or coloring. Fillers help overcome these difficulties.

The hair's porosity determines how much filler is absorbed by the hair shaft. Greater damage allows more filler absorption. Fillers penetrate broken cuticle and

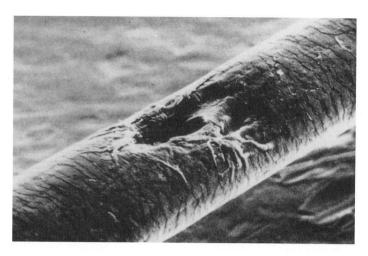

Figure12-6 *"Holes" in the hair shaft, such as this one caused by chlorine bleach, may be treated with fillers to create more even and longer-lasting color.*
(Courtesy: Redken Laboratories, Inc.)

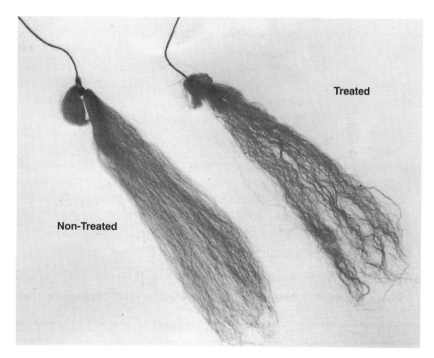

Treated

Non-Treated

Figure12-7 *The above photo shows hair swatches (virgin black) bleached identically, with left swatch without substantive protein. Both swatches were bleached identically demonstrating the compatibility of substantive protein with bleach. You will note the difference in length, brittleness, and strength. The non-protein-treated swatch is harder and rougher than the protein-treated swatch.*

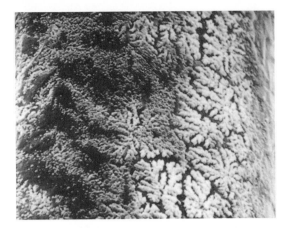 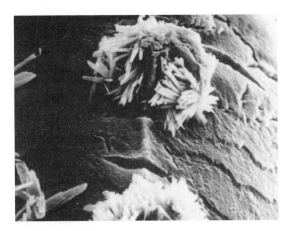

Figure12–8 *Both of these strands of hair have been prebleached and then coated to correct over porosity in preparation for toning.*
(Courtesy: Redken Laboratories, Inc.)

fill "small holes" in the hair. **Fillers** increase the reflective properties of hair and correct excessive porosity. The result is smooth, even coloring with a more intense look.

Fillers are made from protein or fatty materials. They may also contain conditioning agents, direct tints, or other additives (Fig. 12–8).

Toners

Toning prelightened hair to a delicate shade is a successful service in the salon. **Toners** differ from tints only in degree of color saturation. Therefore, toning is actually a technique, rather than a different product type. The same chemistry and safety precautions apply as described for permanent tint applications.

Haircolor Accelerators

There are a variety of products and machines that claim to shorten processing time, eliminate problems, improve the desired results and minimize damage to the hair.

Mechanical Haircolor Processing Machines

Several different machines are sold that claim to shorten the time it takes to process haircolor. One type of machine uses moist heat. These processors usually look something like a sit down hairdryer and must be filled with water. These machines are steamers that heat the water and dispense a hot water vapor inside the hood.

As a general rule, the rate of most chemical reactions increases with an increase in temperature. An increase in temperature of 18°F/10°C doubles the rate of most chemical reactions. This means that a haircolor service processed with a machine at 90°F will process twice as fast as it would at a normal room temperature of 72°F.

Dry heat also shortens processing time and can be applied with a conventional hairdryer or heat lamps. Since dry heat causes evaporation, the hair must be covered with a plastic cap to avoid drying the color mixture. Whenever a plastic cap is used to cover the hair for any chemical process, several small holes should be placed in the cap to allow for the escape of excess heat and any chemical gases that might be formed. Haircolor, or any other chemical, must remain wet in order to process. Haircolor will not process if it is permitted to dry out.

Chemical Haircolor Accelerators

Several different nonirritating, liquid haircolor additives also claim to accelerate the color process and shorten processing time. These nonirritating liquid color additives contain the antioxidant Tocopherol Acetate (Vitamin E), which is claimed to eliminate free radicals and minimize color fading. Other oils are also added that claim to minimize damage and improve the condition of the hair.

These nonirritating, liquid accelerators require the use of a hairdryer. A few drops of the liquid accelerator are added to the color mixture, prior to application. The hair is then covered with a plastic cap and processed under a hairdryer. Remember, even without any additives, haircolor processed at 90°F, will process twice as fast as it would at a normal room temperature of 72°F.

Enzymes

The human body depends on an extremely complex system of chemical reactions that must occur at carefully controlled rates, in order to maintain life. Enzymes are the biological catalysts that control the rates of these reactions. Although enzymes are created by the body, they are not living. Most enzymes are large protein molecules.

Human blood contains the enzyme, catalase, that catalyzes the decomposition of hydrogen peroxide. The bubbling that occurs when 10 volume hydrogen peroxide is applied to a cut is the result of the decomposition of hydrogen peroxide into water and oxygen gas, catalyzed by the enzyme catalase.

Several professional products containing enzymes are sold for use as haircolor additives. These products claim to shorten the processing time and minimize damage to the hair. Although enzymes that aid in the decomposition of hydrogen peroxide should increase the rate of oxidation and shorten the processing time, there is no real evidence that this method is more effective than peroxide or any less damaging to the hair. Enzymes are such large molecules that they are not able to penetrate into the cortex of the hair, where they are needed.

It seems ironic that so many different products and machines are sold to speed up haircolor processing, while the manufacturers of the haircolor deliberately add ingredients to slow the process down. Haircolor is designed to process at a predetermined rate, when mixed and used according to the manufacturer's directions. Without a controlled development of the dyes used in oxidative colors, the color can develop prematurely, prior to penetrating into the cortex of the hair.

Color Removal

There are several methods designed for removing haircolor from a client's hair.

Oil-based haircolor removers lift color from the cuticle. They will not remove dye molecules trapped in the cortex. A large percentage of tinting takes place by staining the cuticle. Therefore, the removers can lighten oxidation tints without causing additional damage to keratin; however, they will not make drastic changes in the color level.

Dye solvents have a greater lightening effect than oil-based removers. These products contain ingredients that breakdown dye molecules. Sodium hydrosulphite, sodium hydrosulphate, and sodium formaldehyde sulphoxylate are the most commonly used products. Peroxides may be used, as well. Dye solvents are alkaline and open the cuticle to allow penetration of active, decolorizing ingredients.

These color removers are strong and irritating to the skin. Some must be mixed with highly corrosive powders and produce irritating vapors. Hairstylists must wear a suitable dust mask, use gloves, and work in a well-ventilated area.

Dye solvents must never be used on hair tinted with metallic "home" coloring products. They are highly incompatible with metallic dyes.

Carefully read and understand manufacturer's instructions before attempting to remove tints. Haircolor removal should only be performed by experienced hairstylists. Improper use can cause serious hair and scalp damage.

NONOXIDATION PERMANENT COLORS

A variety of substances that do not require oxidation will permanently color hair. For example, vegetable dyes have been used for thousands of years. Ancient civilizations didn't have the advantages offered by modern chemistry. They had to rely solely on plant extracts and raw minerals. Science has provided vast improvements in color technology. Nearly all of these archaic techniques have become obsolete.

Henna

Henna is a plant dye that has survived and is occasionally still used today in the henna form. The Egyptian name for this plant is Khenna. Henna is a small, attractive bush with a whitish bark, pale green leaves, and white, fragrant flowers.

The dried, crushed leaves are mixed with water to form a paste. This mixture gives dark, virgin hair an auburn shade. The dye is still used in Arab countries. It is widely believed that the beard of Mohammed was dyed with henna.

Henna is still useful today but has drawbacks. Naturally occurring substances are never pure. Plants contain hundreds of different chemicals necessary for survival and growth. Lawsone, henna dye, is one of the many chemicals found in the henna leaf. It makes up only 1 percent of the leaf.

Tannic acid is also found in the henna leaf. Tannic acid contributes only slightly to hair color. This chemical turns dark upon exposure to light. Unfortunately, tannic acid also increases the stiffness of hair. Henna does not thicken the hair, but it will improve the body of fine hair. Overuse can cause hair to become dry and coarse.

Henna has a strong affinity for the salt bonds in the cortex. This disadvantage causes henna to build up on the hair's surface and in the cortex, thus preventing it from accepting permanent wave applications. The color is not stable and repeated shampooing will cause it to fade slowly. Henna works best on virgin hair. It can give bleached hair a green cast. Although henna is very safe and non-sensitizing, its disadvantages limit its usefulness (Figure 12-9).

Metallic or Metallized Dyes

These color products are not for professional use, but every hairstylist needs to be aware of their properties and use. Metallic colors have existed for as long as vegetable dyes but are rarely used today. The one remaining market is retail, "home

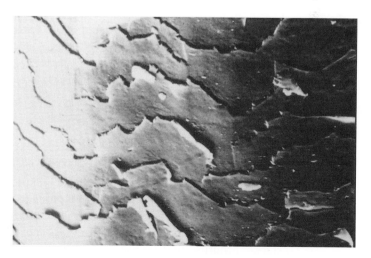

Figure12-9 *Henna attached to the cuticle layer of hair shaft.*
(Courtesy Redken Laboratories, Inc.)

use" color. Metallic dyes are frequently sold as "progressive hair colors" or "color restorers." They do not restore hair to its natural color.

Metallic dyes are naturally occurring salts of lead, silver, copper, and nickel. They are sometimes blended with henna to make **compound dyes.**

Metallic dyes have many disadvantages. Many are toxic if ingested and produce flat, dull metallic-looking colors. They can also produce unexpected or undesirable colors. The cause of green hair is usually copper-based metallic hair colors. Metallic dyes destroy sulfur cross-links in the cortex, leading to hair breakage and loss. The metals interfere with permanent-wave lotions and other professional applications and services. These metals can be absorbed through the skin and reach dangerous levels in the body. Many users report headaches, dermatitis reactions, facial swelling, hair loss and breakage, and even lead poisoning.

Metallic dyes can create many problems for hairstylists. Many professional products used in salons are incompatible with metallic and compound dyes. Metal deposits in the keratin may catalyze violent chemical reactions with oxidizers. For example, hydrogen peroxide can react with metals and melt the hair.

The chemical reactions may be so intense they can result in total, complete, and immediate destruction of the hair.

If you suspect that a client has used metallic or compound dyes, proceed with caution. Strand testing may not provide the information needed to prevent major damage to the hair. It is not recommended that any chemical services, especially those using oxidizers, be performed on hair treated with metallic products.

Usually, the client does not know if the home color contained metal. If the product used was a "restorer" or "progressive" color, it most likely contained metal! All home products should be considered suspect until proven otherwise. Ask the client if he or she remembers the product's name. The client may still have a box, instruction sheet, or original container.

To be sure, test a piece of the client's hair. Instructions for performing such tests are found in *Milady's Standard Textbook of Cosmetology.*

Removal of metallic colors is difficult and not recommended. It is best to cut off the hair that has been treated with metallic products.

HAIR COLORING SAFETY

Since both hair lightening and hair coloring are similar chemical processes, many of the same warnings apply to procedures and products. The high alkalinity and presence of an oxidizer in hair coloring products can cause dermatitis and other problems.

Prior to any application, carefully examine the scalp and hair. Look for signs of scalp irritation, redness, tender or puffy tissue, open sores, excessive dryness, or other skin disorders. Ask the client about problems with previous color applications, (i.e., itchy scalp, sore spots, or irritations). If you suspect scalp problems, advise the client to see a dermatologist before proceeding. Never apply any hair-color to an irritated scalp.

Porosity gradients influence the results. Healthy, virgin hair near the scalp and damaged porous hair ends will cause the color to develop differently. The midstrand is more resistant and requires longer processing times.

Timing and porosity questions can be answered by performing a strand test. Strand tests are important for many reasons. Strand tests help avoid serious prob-lems caused by porosity gradients, damaged hair, temperature changes, and im-proper mixing or application.

Hair nearest the scalp may bleach or lighten more rapidly. This is due to scalp heat, which speeds the chemical reaction. Remember, "the rate of a chem-ical reaction is doubled each time the temperature is raised by 18°F/10°C." Over-lapping color application on previously lightened or tinted hair may result in breakage and excessive damage (Fig. 12-10).

No haircolor process is complete without proper shampooing and rinsing. Alkaline residues become trapped in the keratin. Failure to neutralize these residues causes continued damage. Proper neutralization helps the color maintain its brilliance.

To neutralize residues completely, flush the hair with an organic acid rinse, use a mild, acid shampoo, and condition. Be sure to massage the scalp gently. This will prevent further irritation, if sensitive.

Patch Testing

Professionals are concerned about their client's well-being. Patch testing, or pre-disposition testing, is a critical, important step. Patch tests prevent serious prob-lems and provide proof of precaution and professionalism. Haircolor products are

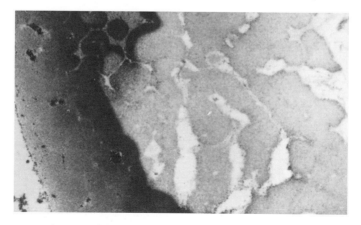

Figure12-10 *This strand has been overbleached. This excessive diffusion of natural pigment will not create the proper foundation for toner development.*
(Courtesy: Redken Laboratories, Inc.)

generally safe if used correctly. However, they are strong alkaline products and contain potent, oxidizing agents. Primary intermediates, modifiers, and other additives may be potential problems, as well. Several common ingredients can cause serious allergic reactions in sensitive individuals (Figs. 12–11 through 12–15).

Symptoms and reactions range from a burning, inflamed scalp to blisters, open sores, and eruptions. Allergic reactions usually begin twelve to fourteen hours after exposure. The first symptoms are usually a painful swelling of the scalp,

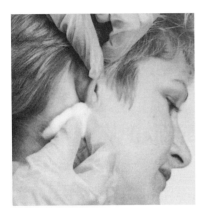

Figure12-11 *Clean area for patch testing.*

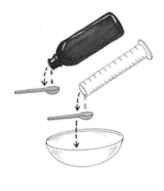

Figure12-12 *Mix tint and peroxide.*

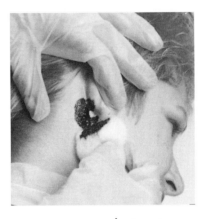

Figure12-13 *Apply tint mixture.*

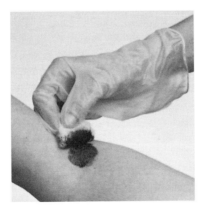

Figure12-14 *A patch test can also be given on the arm.*

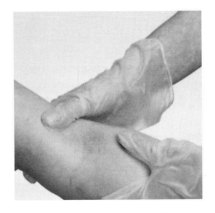

Figure12-15 *A negative skin test will show no sign of inflammation, and an aniline tint may be safely applied.*

> ## CAUTION
>
> This product contains ingredients which may cause skin irritation on certain individuals, and a preliminary test according to the accompanying directions should first be made. This product must not be used for dyeing the eyelashes or eyebrows; to do so may cause blindness.

face, eyes, ears, and neck. Asthma-like breathing difficulties are also sometimes reported.

The ingredients used in tints have improved greatly over the years. The incident rate for such problems has declined. However, even if the chance of a serious reaction is one in 200,000, that one client may walk into your salon.

Federal law requires hairstylists to perform a patch test when using "coal tar dyes." The package warning shown warns you when a patch test is required. Should a client develop a reaction, failure to perform the required test puts the hairstylist in a serious position. The patch test warning statement is found on containers or in manufacturer's instructions:

"Coal tar dyes" also warn against application to the eyebrows and eyelashes. Do not violate these warnings. Always know which products are potential eye hazards. When using these dyes, wear safety glasses and always wash your hands before touching the eye area.

Smart professionals don't take chances. The FDA recommended instructions for performing a patch test are found in Appendix C. Perform the test as directed and record the results on the client's history card. Explain to the client that the law is designed to protect the client. Tell the client that you care about his or her safety. Who would patronize a hairstylist who didn't follow instructions?

Most salons require clients to sign release forms or waivers prior to the application of chemical products. Release forms are invalid if a hairstylist ignores federal law and/or manufacturer's warnings. Don't take chances, protect clients, hairstylists, and salon owners.

Carcinogens, Mutagens, and Teratogens

Substances capable of causing cancer are called *carcinogens* (see Chapter 8). Substances that damage genetic material and affect future generations of children, are called *mutagens*. *Teratogens* adversely affect a developing fetus.

Since 1975, a great controversy has existed over oxidation haircolors. Several scientific studies suggest that certain haircolor ingredients may be dangerous in one or more of the categories mentioned. Since this time, scientific studies have continued to test the safety of haircolors.

Unfortunately, the findings of the studies report conflicting results. No clearcut answer has yet been presented. Therefore, it is concluded that if products are used according to manufacturer's instructions, the products are not likely to be carcinogens, mutagens, or teratogens.

Presently, there is no conclusive evidence that oxidation dyes are too dangerous for salon use.

Don't be careful with just the chemicals you consider harmful. Be careful with all chemicals. Obey the rules of working safely, read and understand the MSDSs, and use the appropriate safety equipment.

Sensitization

Rainbow colored hands are found in many cosmetology schools. Students are often guilty of mishandling semi-permanent and permanent oxidation dyes. Prolonged or repeated exposure to haircolor may cause both irritant contact dermatitis and allergic contact dermatitis.

Overexposure to hair color products and hair bleaches cause over 17 percent of all cosmetic related adverse reactions.[4]

Allergic reactions occur after becoming sensitized to a haircoloring ingredient. Some ingredients in these products are sensitizers.

It may take months or even years to become allergic. This is why client reactions are rare. Once oxidation occurs, the colored dyes are nonsensitizing. Allergic reactions are usually caused by prolonged and/or repeated contact.

Sensitizers pose a special threat to hairstylists. The more often a sensitizing chemical is used, the greater the allergy risk. Generally, an allergic reaction worsens with continued exposure. Eventually, the afflicted person develops *chronic eczema*, an advanced form of allergic dermatitis. The chances of allergy increase if the skin is irritated, broken, or damaged.

REVIEW QUESTIONS

1. Describe the differences among temporary, traditional semi-permanent, long-lasting semi-permanent, and permanent oxidation colors.
2. How do permanent oxidation colors affect melanin?
3. Why do lighteners, semi-permanent colors, and oxidation tints all use ammonia or other alkaline substances in their formulas?
4. Why do semi-permanent dyes last longer than temporary dyes?
5. List the types of ingredients found in oxidation dyes and describe their function.

---

4. U.S. Manufacturers File—1975; information from the FDA Voluntary Cosmetics Regulatory Program.

6. Describe the potential health risks for each of the following: dye solvents, oxidizers, metallic dyes, and oxidation colors.

7. What safety precautions should be used to avoid each of the risks listed in question #6?

8. Describe how to properly perform a patch test.

9. What are sensitizers? Why are they important?

10. How does temperature affect chemical reactions?

DISCUSSION QUESTIONS

1. Discuss the possible consequences of the following situations. In each case, what should the hairstylist do next?

   a. A new client decides to have her hair permanently colored. The hairstylists tells her that she must perform a patch test, but the client is in a hurry and talks her out of doing the federally required test. Early the next morning, the hairstylist receives a call from the client's furious husband. In the middle of the night, the client broke out in a severe rash, her eyes are swollen shut, and she is having great difficulty breathing.

   b. A client wants to have black hair lightened and colored to auburn. The hairstylist fails to do a strand test and the hair comes out medium, dull orange.

   c. A young, client applies hair color at home and ruins the hair. It is dull and metallic gray, instead of a chestnut brown. The client doesn't know what type of color was used. The client wants it fixed before a date in less than five hours. What is the first thing the hairstylist should do? What is the worst thing that could happen if the hair is lightened with peroxide before coloring?

Chapter 13

Permanent Waving

Key Terms

Alkaline waves
Alkanolamines
Aminomethylpropanol and
   monoethanolamine
Ammonium thioglycolate
Croquignole perm
Cysteine
Disulfide bonds
Endothermic waves
Exothermic waves
Glyceryl monothioglycolate
Hydrogen bonds
Modern acid waves
Neutralizers
No ammonia waves
Peptide bonds (or end bonds)
Reduction
Salt bonds
Side bonds
Spiral perm
Thioglycolic acid
Thiol compounds
True acid waves

Learning Objectives

After completing this chapter, you should be able to:

- Relate hair structure to permanent wave chemistry.

- Understand the theory of chemical bonds in hair.

- Describe the action of reducing agents and neutralizers.

- Define hair shape and how it is changed.

- List the different types of waving systems.

- Recognize and avoid typical permanent wave problems.

Probably the greatest tribute to hair's fantastic properties is that it withstands so much abuse. Hair gets brushed, blown, washed, weaved, waved, combed, colored, and curled. But hair can be destroyed!

Permanent waving is an important, practical, and profitable salon service. If done properly, permanents produce beautiful results. If done incorrectly, they may spell disaster.

A detailed step-by-step, guide to proper permanent wave application and neutralization techniques can be found in *Milady's Standard Textbook of Cosmetology*. This chapter will focus on the theory behind the scientific structure of hair and the effects of permanent waving.

You may hear several excuses for why perms fail. Remember, success comes from skill, understanding, and knowledge. Permanent waving involves a scientific process. If you learn the science of permanent waving you will not have failures and won't need excuses.

HAIR STRUCTURE

Permanent waving involves chemical and physical changes within the structure of the hair. Understanding the structure of the hair is essential to understanding permanent waving.

Cuticle

The *cuticle* layer is the tough outer layer that protects the hair from damage. Although a strong cuticle is responsible for resistant hair, the cuticle is not directly involved in permanent waving. The bonds involved in permanent waving are all located within the cortex. The cuticle only interferes with permanent waving because it resists penetration of the permanent waving solution. Alkaline permanent waving solutions soften and swell the hair, which raise the cuticle and permit the solution to penetrate to its target within the cortex.

Cortex

The cortex gives the hair its strength, flexibility, elasticity, and shape. Countless millions of amino acid chains called polypeptides make up the cortex.

Several polypeptide chains cross-link with **disulfide bonds** creating tiny, threadlike fibers that twist around each other to make larger bundles called *micro fibrils*. Dozens of micro fibril, in turn, twist to create larger *macro fibrils*. Finally, macro fibrils intertwine to form fibrils.

The design is much like the high-strength cables used to support suspension bridges. The polypeptide chains found in keratine are both physically and chemically bound together. Millions of these keratinized cells securely bond together to form the cortex. They are covered with a protective cuticle shield, thus creating hair, a super-strength structure with amazing physical characteristics and chemical resistance.

CHEMICAL BONDS

The polypeptide chains are connected by end bonds and cross-linked by side bonds, which form the fibers and structure of hair. These chemical bonds hold the hair in its natural shape and are responsible for the incredible strength and elasticity of human hair.

Peptide Bonds (End Bonds)

Proteins are made of long chains of amino acids linked together, end to end, like pop beads. The chemical bonds that link amino acids together are called **peptide** (**PEP**-tyd) **bonds** or **end bonds**. Long chains of amino acids, linked by peptide bonds, are called polypeptides. Proteins are long, coiled, complex polypeptides made of many different amino acids.

Although different amino acids have different structures, all amino acids have an amino end and an acid end. The amino end contains an amine group (-NH_2), which is alkaline, like ammonia (NH_3). The acid end contains a carboxylic acid (COOH), which is acidic. Peptide bonds join the amino end of one amino acid with the acid end of another amino acid to form a polypeptide chain.

Polypeptides, the smallest individual strands in keratin, are polymers of amino acids. When two or more amino acids chemically join, they are called *peptides*. Polypeptides are long chains of peptides. Polypeptide chains may contain over 8,000 amino acids. These bonds are the major, binding force for all protein structures, including hair.

Peptide bonds are the strongest chemical bonds in the hair, but if even a few are broken, the hair becomes weak and damaged. If more peptide bonds are broken and remain broken, the hair will completely break off. Luckily, under normal circumstances, peptide bonds are not involved in the chemical action of salon services.

Side Bonds

The cortex is made of millions of polypeptide chains, which are cross-linked by three different types of **side bonds**: disulfide bonds, salt bonds, and hydrogen bonds. Altering these side bonds is what makes wet sets, thermal styling, permanent waving, and chemical hair relaxing possible.

Hair is an insoluble, *complex protein*. Cross-linking a coiled, simple protein (polypeptide) creates complex proteins. This is like placing tiny bridges between the coils of a spring. The bridges make the spring stronger and more rigid.

Disulfide Bonds (Side Bonds)

Disulfide side bonds are formed between two **cysteine** (**SIS**-tuh-een) amino acids, located on neighboring polypeptide chains. A **disulfide bond** joins two sulfur atoms, one from each of the two neighboring cysteine amino acids. A disulfide side bond joins a cysteine sulfur atom on one polypeptide chain with a second cysteine sulfur atom on a neighboring polypeptide chain. Disulfide bonds are weaker than peptide bonds but much stronger than hydrogen or salt bonds.

Disulfide bonds are strong, covalent side bonds that are not broken by heat or water. Although fewer disulfide bonds exist than hydrogen or salt bonds, disulfide bonds are much stronger and account for about one-third of the hair's overall strength. As we will soon see, the chemical and physical changes in disulfide bonds make permanent waving and chemical hair relaxing possible.

Almost all the cystine in hair is found in the cortex and cuticle layers. The extremely hard cuticle contains the highest percentage of cystine.

Salt Bonds (Side Bonds)

Salt bonds are relatively weak ionic side bonds. You should remember from Chapter 9 that ionic bonds are the result of an attraction between opposite electrical charges. Within the structure of the hair, a salt bond occurs when the negative charge of an amino acid on one polypeptide chain is attracted to the positive charge of an amino acid on a neighboring polypeptide chain. Salt bonds are much weaker and less resistant than disulfide bonds. Salt bonds are weakened by water and easily broken by alkaline solutions. Salt bonds are far weaker than disulfide bonds, but there are so many more salt bonds, they account for about one-third of the hair's total strength. Salt bonds are affected greatly by changes in pH level. At high pH levels, an amino acid may alter its charge from positive to negative. Then there are two negatively charged amino acids side by side. The negatively charged amino acids will repel each other and push apart. This is why hair swells and the cuticle lifts when alkaline solutions are applied.

Hydrogen Bonds (Side Bonds)

Hydrogen bonds are a special type of ionic bond. Within the structure of hair, a hydrogen side bond occurs when a hydrogen atom, from the acid portion of an amino acid on one polypeptide chain, is attracted to an oxygen atom, in the acid portion of an amino acid on a neighboring polypeptide chain. Although individual hydrogen bonds are weak, there are so many of them in the hair that they account for about one-third of the hair's total strength.

Hydrogen bonds are weaker and less resistant than all other bonds in the hair. Hydrogen bonds are easily broken, simply by wetting the hair with water, and are reformed when the hair is dried.

1. **Straight Hair**
   (Showing position of H and S bonds.)

2. **Hair Softened by Water.**
   (H bonds are broken).

3. **Hair Wound On Rollers.**
   (S bonds stretched into waved positions.)

4. **Hair After Proper Drying.**
   (H bonds reformed into waved positions.)

5. **Hair After Brushing Out Into Set.**
   (Waves held only by H bonds.) Hair is sprayed with moisture-repellent barrier.

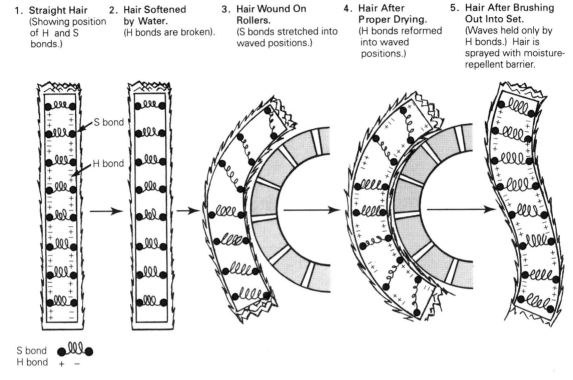

Figure 13–1 *Changes in hair cortex during wet setting.*

When hair absorbs water, the shaft swells. This happens because water interferes with the hydrogen bonds between amino acids. The amino acids form hydrogen bonds with the water instead of with each other. When the hydrogen bonds between the amino acids break, the polypeptide chains push apart, causing the hair shaft to swell. A wet set is an example of a physical change that results from breaking and reforming the hydrogen bonds within the hair. Wetting the hair breaks the hydrogen bonds and permits the hair to be stretched and wrapped on rollers. Drying the hair removes the water and reforms the hydrogen bonds in their new shape. These changes are only temporary. As soon as the hair is wet or exposed to high humidity, it will revert to its original shape (Fig. 13–1).

Thermal styling with hair dryers, curling irons, and pressing combs also break hydrogen bonds within the hair, just like a wet set. These styles involve a physical change and the results are only temporary. The hair will revert to its original shape as soon as it is wet.

PERMANENT WAVING

Permanent waving is a two-step process involving a physical and a chemical change. The first part of any perm is the physical change caused by wrapping the hair on the rods. The second part involves the chemical changes caused by the perm solution and the neutralizer.

The Perm Wrap

In permanent waving, the size and type of curl is determined by the size of the rods and the type of wrapping method. Permanent waving solution, by itself, does not cause the hair to curl any more than water causes a wet set to curl. Permanent waving solution simply softens the hair, allowing it to conform to the shape in which it was wrapped. As long as a perm is processed correctly, what you wrap is what you get.

The first step in any permanent is wrapping it in the desired shape. If you have ever set someone's hair on perm rods and let it dry, you have completed the physical part of a permanent. Aside from any differences in wrapping, the major difference between a wet set and a permanent wave is in the types of side bonds that are broken. In a perm wrap, just as in a wet set, wetting the hair with water breaks the hydrogen bonds and permits the hair to be wrapped in the desired shape. A perm wrap is essentially a wet set on perm rods instead of rollers (Fig. 13–2).

1. **Straight Hair**
   (Both H and S bonds in straight positions.)

2. **Hair Wound On Rods and Softened by Shampooing and Cold Wave Solutions.**
   (H bonds and nearly all S bonds broken.)

3. **Hair After Neutralizing.**
   (Some H Bonds and many S bonds reformed.)

4. **Hair On Rollers After Proper Drying.**
   (Most H bonds reformed as well as S bonds.)

5. **Hair After Unwinding.**
   (Original S bonds stretched into waved positions.)

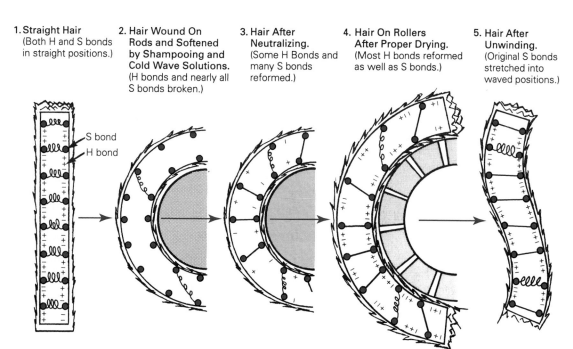

Figure 13-2 *Changes in hair cortex during permanent waving.*

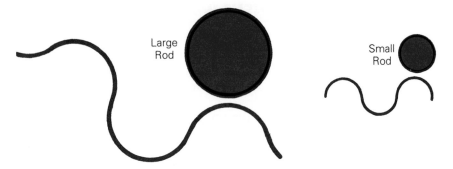

Figure 13-3 *The size of the rod determines the size of the curl. A small rod gives a tight curl and a large rod gives a loose curl.*

All other things being equal, the size of the perm rod determines the size of the curl. Small rods produce small curls and large rods produce large curls (Fig. 13–3). Wrapping the hair on small rods increases the tension, which increases the amount of curl. Although tension produces the curl, too much tension, especially in one spot, can mark or break the hair. Keep the hair wet while wrapping, and always wrap with uniform, even tension.

Croquignole Perm Wrap

In a **croquignole (KROH**-ken-ohl) **perm** wrap, the hair is wrapped from the ends to the scalp in overlapping, concentric layers (Figs. 13–4 and 13–5). Because the hair is wrapped at an angle perpendicular to the length of the rod, each new layer of hair is wrapped on top of the previous layer, as the rod is wrapped toward the scalp. Since the effective size of the rod increases with each new overlapping

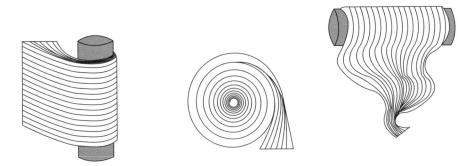

Figure 13-4 *In a croquignole perm, each layer of hair is wrapped on top of the preceding layer, which makes the effective size of the rod larger as the hair gets closer to the scalp. The resulting curl is larger at the scalp and tighter at the ends.*

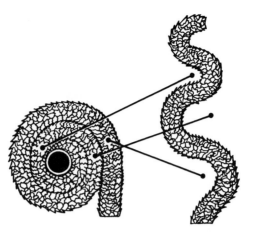

Figure 13-5 *Hair croquignole wound on a rod, giving a larger curl on the top layer.*

layer, this wrapping method produces a tighter curl at the ends and a larger curl at the scalp. Longer, thicker hair increases this effect.

Spiral Perm Wrap

Most **spiral perms** are wrapped from the ends to the scalp, although depending on the rods used, some may be wrapped from the scalp to the ends. The difference should not affect the finished curl. In a spiral perm wrap, the hair is wrapped at an angle other than perpendicular to the length of the rod. The angle at which the hair is wrapped causes the hair to spiral along the length of the rod, like the grip on a tennis racquet (Figs. 13–6 and 13–7).

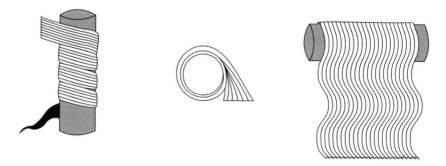

Figure 13-6 *In a spiral perm, each layer of hair is wrapped against the rod, which makes the effective size of the rod the same throughout the length of the hair strand. The resulting curl is the same size from the scalp to the ends.*

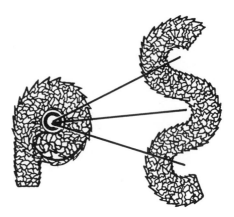

Figure 13-7 *Hair spiral wound on small rod, giving tight, even wave.*

In a spiral perm wrap, each layer of hair partially overlaps the preceding layer. As long as the angle remains constant, any overlapping will be uniform along the length of the rod and the entire strand of hair. Since the effective size of the rod remains constant along the entire strand of hair, this wrapping method produces a uniform curl from the scalp to the ends. Longer, thicker hair will benefit most from this type of perm wrap.

THE CHEMISTRY OF PERMANENT WAVING

Permanent wave solutions cause the hair to undergo a chemical change. Strong, alkaline substances cause disulfide bonds to break. Alkaline solutions also make ionic bonds repel each other, instead of attract. This will make the hair shaft swell and lift the cuticle.

Alkaline reducing agents have a high pH. These highly alkaline solutions open the cuticle and allow penetration into the cortex. At a pH level of 9, the hair shaft can swell up to twice its normal diameter.

Alkaline permanent waving solution softens and swells the hair, which raises the cuticle and permits the solution to penetrate to its target within the cortex (Figs. 13–8 through 13–11). Once in the cortex, permanent waving solution breaks the disulfide bonds by a chemical reaction called **reduction**. You should remember from Chapter 9 that a reduction reaction involves either the addition of hydrogen or the removal of oxygen. The reduction reaction in permanent waving is due to the addition of hydrogen.

A disulfide bond joins two sulfur atoms. A disulfide bond joins a sulfur atom on one polypeptide chain, with a second sulfur atom on a neighboring polypeptide chain. Permanent waving solution breaks a disulfide bond by adding a "free" hydrogen atom to each of the sulfur atoms in the disulfide bond. The sulfur atoms

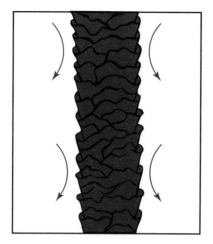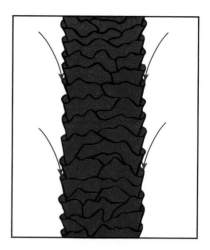

Figure 13-8 *Action of wetting agents on hair-waving solutions. Solution with wetting agent, right, allows penetration while solution without, left, does not.*

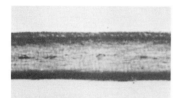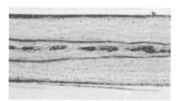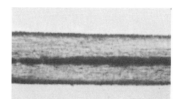

Figure 13-9 *Hair in ammonium thioglycolate solution (pH 9.4) for 5 minutes. Slight swelling of imbrications.*

Figure 13-10 *The same hair in ammonium thioglycolate (pH 12.5) for 5 minutes; severe swelling of cortex.*

Figure 13-11 *The same hair in neutral waving solution (pH 7.5) for 5 minutes.*

attach to the free hydrogen atoms, from the permanent waving solution, and break their attachment to each other (Fig. 13–12). Once the disulfide bond is broken, the polypeptide chains are able to slip into their new curled shape.

The reducing agents used in permanent waving solutions are **thiol (THY**-ohl) **compounds.** They are also called mercaptans and are commonly referred to simply as *thio* (**THY**-oh). **Thioglycolic** (thy-oh-**GLY**-kohl-ic) **acid** ($HSCH_2COOH$) is the most common. Thioglycolic acid provides the free hydrogen ions (H^+) that cause the reduction reaction in permanent waving solutions and break the disulfide bonds.

The strength of the permanent waving solution is determined by the concentration of thioglycolic acid. Stronger perms have a higher concentration of

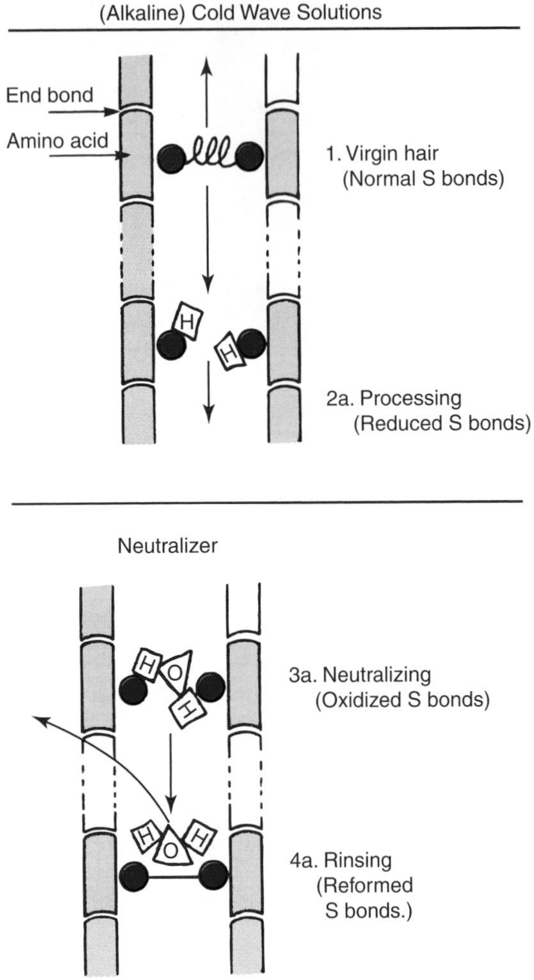

(Alkaline) Cold Wave Solutions

End bond

Amino acid

1. Virgin hair
(Normal S bonds)

2a. Processing
(Reduced S bonds)

Neutralizer

3a. Neutralizing
(Oxidized S bonds)

4a. Rinsing
(Reformed
S bonds.)

Figure 13-12 *Chemistry of cold waving.*

thioglycolic acid and a greater number of free hydrogen atoms. When more free hydrogen atoms are available, more disulfide bonds can be broken.

Since strong, thick, coarse hair contains more disulfide bonds than fine, thin hair, it needs a strong solution with a high concentration of thioglycolic acid. And since fine, weak, or chemically damaged hair contains fewer disulfide bonds than thick, coarse hair, it only needs a weak solution with a low concentration of thioglycolic acid. Strong permanent waving solutions contain higher concentrations of thioglycolic acid and are able to break more disulfide bonds. Weak permanent waving solutions contain lower concentrations of thioglycolic acid and break fewer disulfide bonds. A strong solution can break more disulfide bonds

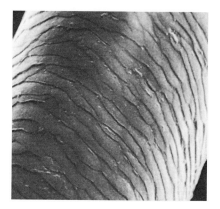

Figure 13-13 *Normal cuticle structure.*
(Courtesy: Gillette Company Research Institute, Rockville, Maryland)

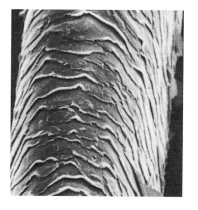

Figure 13-14 *Resistant hair.*
(Courtesy: Gillette Company Research Institute, Rockville, Maryland)

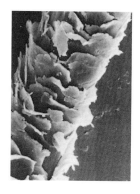

Figure 13-15 *Tinted hair with high porosity.*
(Courtesy: Gillette Company Research Institute, Rockville, Maryland)

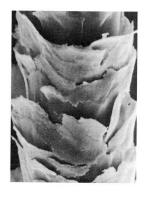

Figure 13-16 *Damaged cuticle with high porosity*
(Courtesy: Gillette Company Research Institute, Rockville, Maryland)

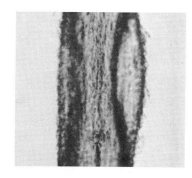

Figure 13-17 *Hair showing area of greater porosity. When cold waving, this would require preconditioning treatment to avoid this type of damage from thio.*

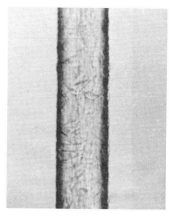

Figure 13-18 *Lightened hair after shampooing and rinsing*

than a weak solution. The strength of the perm solution should correspond to the strength of the hair.

Thioglycolic acid is an acid, and since acids don't penetrate into the cortex, it's necessary for the manufacturers to add an alkali. The addition of ammonia to thioglycolic acid makes a new chemical called **ammonium thioglycolate** (uh-**MOH**-nee-um thy-oh-**GLY**-kohl-ayt) ($HSCH_2COOHNH_4$). Ammonium thioglycolate is the reducing agent in most alkaline permanent waves.

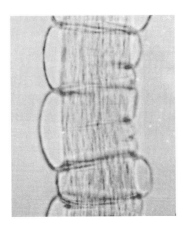

Figure 13-19 *Same hair after 5 minutes in ammonium thioglycolate (pH 9.4). Gross swelling of cuticle has detached scales from hair shaft.*

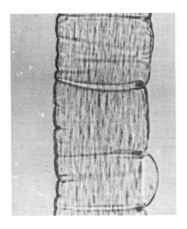

Figure 13-20 *After 8 minutes in "thio" cold-waving solution. Cortex has swelled excessively. Severe damage occurs when using alkaline-waving solutions on lightened hair.*

The degree of alkalinity (pH) contributes a second component to the overall strength of permanent waving solution. Hair with a strong, resistant cuticle layer needs the additional swelling and penetration provided by a more alkaline permanent waving solution. Fine hair or hair with a damaged cuticle layer is easily penetrated and would be damaged less by a permanent waving solution with a lower pH. The alkalinity of the perm solution should correspond to the strength and resistance of the cuticle layer.

TYPES OF PERMANENT WAVES

The Machine Wave

In 1905, Charles Nessler invented the first permanent waving machine. The hair was wrapped on metal rods that were heated by an electrical current from Nessler's machine. Twenty-six years later, other machines were developed that used pre-heated clamps that were placed over the wound curls. Although these methods worked, they damaged the hair and were dangerous for the client.

Alkaline Waves or Cold Waves

The first **alkaline waves** were developed in 1941 and relied on the same ammonium thioglycolate (ATG) that is still used in today's alkaline waves. Since alkaline waves could be given at room temperature without added heat, they also became known as cold waves. Most alkaline waves have a pH between 9.0 and 9.6. The terms *alkaline wave, cold wave,* and *thio* are interchangeable.

These high pH levels cause the hair shaft to swell, lifting the cuticle. Proper measuring and mixing of solution is very important. Hair will begin to dissolve above a pH value of 10. Serious errors can result from failure to follow the manufacturer's instructions. Never use any product until you read and understand the instructions.

True Acid Waves

The first **true acid waves** were introduced in the early '70s. True acid waves have a pH between 4.5 and 7.0 and use **glyceryl monothioglycolate** (GMTG) (**GLIS**-ur-yl mon-oh-thy-oh-**GLY**-koh-layt) as the primary reducing agent. Although a lower pH causes significantly less damage, acid waves process more slowly and do not produce as firm a curl as alkaline waves. Most true acid waves require the added heat of a hair dryer to accelerate processing (Fig. 13–21 and Appendix E).

Although acid waves don't swell the hair as much as alkaline waves, all permanent waves cause the hair to swell. Some swelling is essential to the chemical action of any permanent wave. Since alkaline solutions swell the hair, we expect alkaline waves to swell the hair. Since acidic solutions contract the hair, how can a true acid wave with a pH of less than 7.0 cause the hair to swell?

In Chapter 9, we learned that the average pH of hair is 5.0. So, although a pH of 7.0 is neutral on the pH scale, a pH of 5.0 is neutral for hair. Since every step in the pH scale represents a tenfold change in pH, a pH of 7.0 is one hundred times more alkaline than the pH of hair. Even pure water will damage the hair and cause it to swell.

Modern Acid Waves

In order to process at room temperature and produce a firmer curl, the strength and pH of acid waves has increased steadily over the years. Most of the acid waves

CHECKING POROSITY

More than ever, today's advanced products require special skills and training. Changing permanent waving techniques are good examples. Permanent wave success often depends on choosing the right product for a client's hair. The porosity of the hair is an important factor in this decision.

Simply described, porosity is the hair's ability to absorb liquids. Virgin hair cuticles form a tight, liquid-resistant barrier. This protective shield works much like a suit of armor.

Normal and resistant hair is not very porous. Both are resistant to chemicals and moisture, but to differing degrees. Once damaged by environmental, mechanical, or chemical factors, the cuticle no longer makes a tight shield. Damage to the cuticle makes it easier for liquids to penetrate. The greater the cuticle damage, the higher the porosity.

Evaluate the extent of damage and degree of porosity before each service. These observations help you make recommendations about salon services and home maintenance care.

Porosity is best evaluated on clean, dry hair. Check different parts of the head (i.e., the front hair line, behind the ear, and in the crown areas). Gently slide a single strand of hair between your fingers, from the tip towards the scalp. Normal to resistant hair feels smooth and silky. Roughness indicates a raised cuticle. The more damaged the hair, the rougher the texture. Using a few dozen strands, repeat the test several times.

As you gain practice, it becomes easy to recognize hair that is resistant, normal, damaged, or very damaged. Make a habit of feeling hair. You will quickly become an expert at determining other properties, such as density, texture, thickness, etc.

found in today's salons have a pH between 7.8 and 8.2, which means they aren't really acidic. **Modern acid waves** are not true acid waves but are actually *acid-balanced waves*. Because of their slightly higher pH, modern acid waves process at room temperature and do not require the added heat of a hair dryer. Modern acid waves also process quicker and produce firmer curls than true acid waves.

Glyceryl monothioglycolate (GMTG) is the primary reducing agent in all acid waves. All acids waves have three components: permanent waving solution, activator, and neutralizer. The activator tube contains GMTG and must be added to the permanent waving solution immediately prior to use. Although GMTG is the primary reducing agent, it is not usually the only reducing agent. The permanent waving solution in most modern acid-balanced waves usually also contains ammonium thioglycolate (ATG) (Fig. 13–21 and Appendix E).

Although the low pH of acid waves may seem ideal, repeated exposure to GMTG is known to cause allergic sensitivity in both hairstylists and clients.

The chances of irritant and allergic contact dermatitis are lessened if scalp and skin contact is limited.

Always wear gloves while using permanent waving lotions, especially low pH products. Watch clients closely for signs of allergy or irritation. If problems develop, suggest they see a dermatologist.

SELF-HEATING PERMS

Exothermic Waves

An exothermic chemical reaction releases heat to its surroundings. **Exothermic** (ek-soh-**THUR**-mik) **waves** involve an exothermic chemical reaction that releases heat and causes the permanent waving solution to become hot.

All exothermic waves have three components: permanent waving solution, activator, and neutralizer. The activator tube contains an oxidizing agent (usually hydrogen peroxide) that must be added to the permanent waving solution immediately prior to use (Fig. 13-21 and Appendix E). Mixing an oxidizer

TYPES OF PERMS

ACID WAVING LOTION	ALKALINE WAVING LOTION	EXOTHERMIC WAVING LOTION	NO AMMONIA LOW THIO WAVING LOTION
Ammonium Thioglycolate	Ammonium Thioglycolate	Ammonium Thioglycolate	Ethanolamine Thioglycolate
Ammonium Hydroxide	Ammonium Hydroxide	Ammonium Hydroxide	Mercaptamine
Diammonium Dithioglycolate	Diammonium Dithioglycolate	Ammonium Bicarbonate	Ethanolamine
DMDM Hydrantoin	Ammonium Bicarbonate	Dimethicone	Urea
Nonoxynol-15	Nonoxynol-15	Nonoxynol-15	Nonoxynol-15
Polyquaternium-10	Polyquaternium-28	Quaternium-75	Propylene Glycol
Sodium Borate	Glycerin	Silica	Glycerine
Fragrance	Fragrance	Fragrance	Fragrance
Water	Water	Water	Water
		EDTA	EDTA

ACTIVATOR		ACTIVATOR	
Glycerin		Hydrogen Peroxide	
Glyceryl Thioglycolate		Dicetyldimonium Chloride	
		Dimethicone	
		Phosphoric Acid	
		Silica	
		Water	

NEUTRALIZER	NEUTRALIZER	NEUTRALIZER	NEUTRALIZER
Hydrogen Peroxide	Hydrogen Peroxide	Hydrogen Peroxide	Hydrogen Peroxide
Dicetyldimonium Chloride	Dicetyldimonium Chloride	Sodium Phosphate	Dicetyldimonium Chloride
Dimethicone	Dimethicone	Polyquaternium-6	Dimethicone
Phosphoric Acid	Phosphoric Acid	Phosphoric Acid	Phosphoric Acid
Silica	Silica	Water	Silica
Water	Water		Water

Figure 13-21 A list of common permanent waving ingredients, listed in order for easy comparison.

with the permanent waving solution causes a rapid release of heat and an increase in the temperature. The increase in temperature increases the rate of the chemical reaction, which shortens the processing time. The rate of a chemical reaction doubles with an increase in temperature of 18°F/10°C.

Endothermic Waves

An endothermic chemical reaction absorbs heat from its surroundings. **Endothermic** (end-oh-**THUR**-mik) **waves** require heat from a hair dryer and will not process properly at room temperature. Most true acid waves are endothermic and require the additional heat provided by a hair dryer. Remember that heat increases the rate of any chemical reaction.

No Ammonia Waves

Just like haircolor and hair lighteners, **no ammonia waves** use **alkanolamines** (al-kan-all-**AM**-eenz) (Chapter 11, Color and Hair Lightening) to replace ammonia and are gaining in popularity because of their low odor. These large, organic molecules contain carbon and are not as volatile as ammonia, so there is little odor associated with their use. **Aminomethylpropanol** (AMP) (uh-**MEE**-noh-meth-yl-pro-pan-all), and **monoethanolamine** (MEA) (mahn-oh-**ETH**-an-all-am-een) are examples of organic alkalis that are used in permanent waving solutions instead of ammonia (Fig. 13–21 and Appendix E).

Although ammonia has an offensive smell, it may actually be better suited to permanent waving and less damaging to the hair. Ammonia (NH_3) is a volatile, inorganic molecule that evaporates very quickly as a gas. As the ammonia evaporates, the pH drops. That means that the pH decreases during processing. An ammonia alkaline wave that starts out at a pH of 9.6 quickly drops to about 8.2 during processing. A high pH is not necessary once the cuticle is raised and the hair has been fully saturated. It's far less damaging if the remainder of the processing is at a lower pH.

Alkanolamines evaporate slowly, which is why they don't smell. The no ammonia waves remain at the same pH throughout the entire processing time. Although the no ammonia waves may start out at a lower pH, they will remain at the same pH throughout the entire processing time. Even though alkanolamines may not smell as strong as ammonia, they can be every bit as alkaline. Ammonia free does not mean free of damage.

PERMANENT WAVE PROCESSING

The strength of a permanent wave is due to the concentration of the reducing agent and the pH of the solution. The amount of processing is determined by the strength of the permanent waving solution. If weak permanent waving solution is used on coarse hair, there may not be enough hydrogen atoms to break the necessary number of disulfide bonds, no matter how long the solution processes. But the same weak solution may be perfect for fine hair with fewer disulfide bonds. On the other hand, a strong solution, which releases many hydrogen atoms, may be perfect for coarse hair, but extremely damaging to fine hair. The amount of processing is determined by the strength of the solution, not necessarily how long it processes.

Although baking a cake twice as long will cook it twice as much, processing a permanent wave twice as long, does not necessarily mean processing it twice as much. The rate at which a cake bakes is uniform over time because energy is added to the oven during baking. A cake baked for thirty minutes will cook twice as much as one baked for fifteen minutes.

Unlike baking a cake, the rate of most chemical reactions is not uniform and diminishes rapidly. In most chemical reactions, the amount of chemical activity is determined by the concentration of the reactants. The reactants only react once and are "used up" as they form products. So, as the concentration of reactants diminishes, so does the rate of the chemical reaction. In permanent waving, most of the processing takes place as soon as the solution penetrates the hair within the first five to ten minutes (Fig. 13–22). The additional time involved in processing allows the polypeptide chains to shift into their new configuration.

This means that if the hair is overprocessed, it probably happened within the first five to ten minutes and a weaker permanent waving solution should have been used. This also means that if the hair is not sufficiently processed within the first five to ten minutes, it probably never will be and a stronger solution, or a more thorough saturation of solution, may be needed.

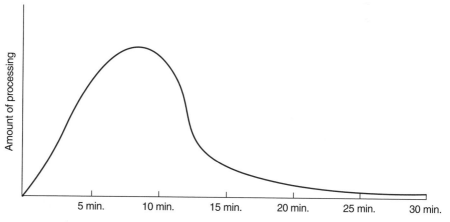

Figure 13–22 *The graph shows that the rate of most chemical reactions is not uniform over time. The rate of reaction begins slowly until the chemicals penetrate the hair, then drops sharply as the reactants are "used up" and converted to products. Most chemical reactions have very little chemical activity after 20 minutes.*

Thorough saturation of the hair is essential to proper processing in all permanent waves, but especially on resistant hair. Regardless of the strength of the solution, resistant hair may not become completely saturated with just one application of waving solution. Continue to apply solution slowly until the hair is completely saturated. If the hair is not saturated sufficiently, it will not process properly. If the curl development is not sufficient after ten minutes and the hair is not wet and completely saturated, reapplication of the waving solution may be necessary.

Stronger solutions will process the hair more, but processing the hair more does not necessarily mean more curl. A properly processed permanent wave should break and rebuild approximately 50 percent of the hair's disulfide bonds. If too many disulfide bonds are broken, the hair may not have enough strength to hold the desired curl. Weak hair equals a weak curl.

Contrary to what many believe, over processed hair is not overly curly. If too many disulfide bonds are broken, the hair will be too weak to hold a firm curl. Over processed hair usually has a weak curl or may be completely straight. Since the hair at the scalp is usually stronger than the ends, overprocessed hair is usually curlier at the scalp, and straighter at the ends. If the hair is overprocessed, processing it more will make it straighter.

Underprocessed hair is exactly the opposite. If too few disulfide bonds are broken, the hair will not be sufficiently softened and it will be unable to hold the desired curl. Underprocessed hair usually has a weak curl, but it may also be straight. Since the hair at the scalp is usually stronger than the ends, underprocessed hair is usually straighter at the scalp, and curlier at the ends (Fig. 13–32). If the hair is underprocessed, processing it more will make it curlier.

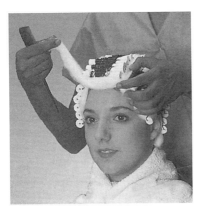

Figure 13-23 *Hairline protected by cotton strips or neutralizing band.*

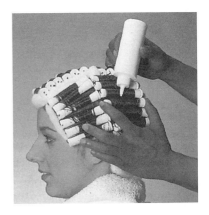

Figure 13-24 *Application of waving lotion.*

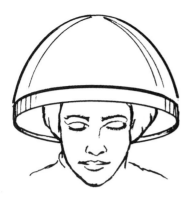

Figure 13-25 *Placing a client under a pre-heated dryer accelerates processing.*

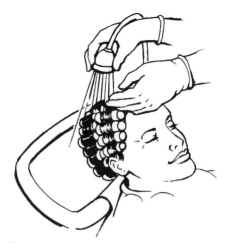

Figure 13-26 *Thorough rinsing with warm water is essential to remove all traces of excess cold-waving solution from the hair.*

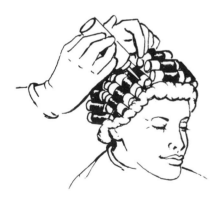

Figure 13-27 *When rinsing is completed, the neutralizer is carefully applied to the hair on the rods.*

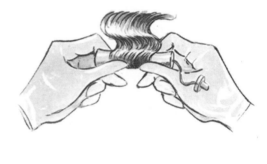

Figure 13-28 *Method of taking a test curl to determine processing time.*

It is important to develop a foolproof system for timing permanent waving services. Use a timer with an alarm. Check the wave development progress often. This improves the quality of service and will help avoid overprocessing. Improper timing may cause delayed action chemical burns that might not appear until several hours later.

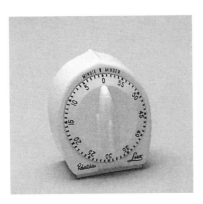

Figure 13-29 *Proper timing is essential when performing a perm service.*

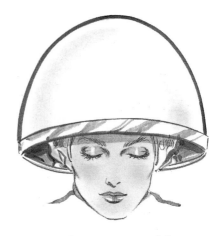

Figure 13-30 *The temperature of the perming process can have an important bearing on effective waving.*

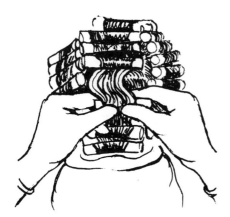

Figure 13-31 *Improper winding technique can cause perm failure.*

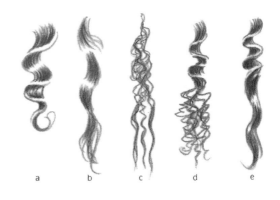

a   b   c   d   e

Figure 13-32 *Curl results: a. good results; b. underprocessed curl; c. over-processed curl; d. porous ends; e. improper winding.*

NEUTRALIZATION

Proper neutralization performs two important functions. A neutralizer gets its name because it neutralizes any waving solution that remains in the hair. Neutralization also rebuilds the disulfide bonds that were broken by the waving solution.

The name **neutralizer** is not accurate because the chemical reaction involved is oxidation. Neutralizers are actually oxidizers. The most common neutralizer is hydrogen peroxide. Concentrations vary between 5 volume (1.5 percent) and 10 volume (3 percent). Other types of neutralizers are sodium bromate ($NaBrO_3$), and sodium perborate ($NaBO_3$). Non-peroxide neutralizers are more stable than peroxide, but they aren't more effective or less damaging.

Although the neutralizer will neutralize any remaining waving solution, the chemical reaction involved is oxidation. Remember that exothermic waves get hot when an oxidizer is mixed with the waving solution, and oxidation reactions also lighten hair color, especially at a high pH. To avoid scalp irritation and unwanted lightening of hair color, always rinse the hair for at least five minutes, prior to applying the neutralizer.

After a thorough rinsing and before applying the neutralizer, most manufacturers recommend that the hair be blotted with towels to remove excess moisture. Excess water left in the hair dilutes the neutralizer and prevents uniform saturation.

Neutralization also rebuilds the disulfide bonds that were broken during processing. You should remember from earlier in this chapter that the waving solution breaks disulfide bonds by adding hydrogen atoms to the sulfur atoms in the disulfide bond. Neutralization rebuilds the disulfide bonds by removing those extra hydrogen atoms.

The hydrogen atoms in the disulfide bonds are so strongly attracted to the extra oxygen atom in the neutralizer that they release their bond with the sulfur atoms and join with the oxygen (Fig. 13–12). Each oxygen atom attaches to two hydrogen atoms to rebuild one disulfide bond and make one molecule of water ($H_2 + O \rightarrow H_2O$). The water is removed in the final rinse and the sulfur atoms form new disulfide bonds in their new curled position.

When the neutralizer removes the extra hydrogen atoms, each sulfur atom forms a new bond with its nearest neighboring sulfur atom. This is not the same pair that was originally bonded, but a newly created pair, which will hold the hair in the new shape (Fig 13–33).

The neutralizer in a permanent wave performs the same function as a hairdryer does in a wet set. In a wet set, the hydrogen bonds are broken by water. When the water is removed by drying, the hydrogen bonds are reformed. The hairdryer simply speeds up the drying process, which makes the hair dry quickly. The hairdryer isn't needed in a wet set. Given enough time, the hair would dry on its own. Once the hair is dry, the hydrogen bonds are reformed.

When neutralizing a permanent wave, the neutralizer adds oxygen to the hair and rebuilds the disulfide bonds. The neutralizer provides a high concentration of liquid oxygen, which simply speeds up the process and rebuilds the disulfide bonds quickly. At one time, neutralizer was called instant neutralizer.

Once a permanent wave is processed, rinsed, and blotted, it's ready for neutralization. Although liquid neutralizer is usually used, it's not really necessary. Neutralization can take place naturally without a liquid neutralizer. If the hair has

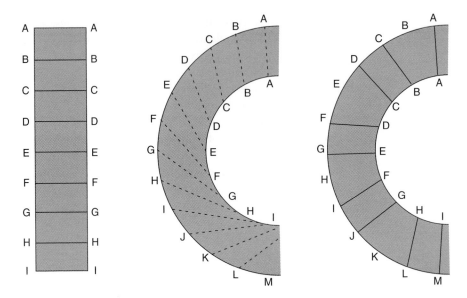

Figure 13-33 Diagram shows the tension placed on the side bonds when hair is stretched around the perm rod. The broken side bonds are then reformed, into their new shape, as different pairs.

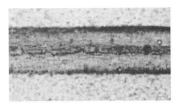

Figure 13-34 Hair in cold-wave neutralizer (pH 3.0). Note droplets of conditioner in o/w type.

been properly processed, rinsed, and blotted, it can be left to neutralize on its own. Given enough time, the hair draws oxygen from the atmosphere, which performs the same function as the oxygen in the liquid neutralizer. Once the hair is dry, neutralization is complete. It's really not any different than letting a wet set dry on its own without a hairdryer.

All safety precautions previously described for oxidizers should be used. There are many different methods for applying and neutralizing permanent wave products. It is important to follow manufacturer's instructions and the rules of working safely. This is especially true for perm rinsing and neutralizing.

Proper rinsing and neutralization are vital to the success of the permanent wave. Reducing agent is found deep within the cortex. The waving process can only be halted by completely rinsing and neutralizing the hair. Improper neutralization may cause a 20 percent loss of hair strength. Scalp burns can also result from improper rinsing and neutralization. The client may not feel pain until several hours later (Figs 13–24 and 13–25).

Use only the manufacturer-recommended neutralizer with the perm lotion. Never mix brands or systems.

Powdered neutralizers contain oxidizers, usually sodium bromate or sodium perborate. Follow all safety precautions previously described for powdered oxidizers. Wear a dust mask while mixing or measuring these products and work in a properly-ventilated area. Be sure to wear safety glasses and gloves, as these chemicals are potential eye and skin hazard.

Caution: Serious accidents can occur when hairstylists mistakenly use neutralizers instead of water as permanent wave lotion rinses. Intense heat can be generated if the hair is not first rinsed thoroughly with water. This error may seriously burn a client's scalp.

WAVE SAFETY

Ammonium thioglycolate (ATG) and ammonia are responsible for the odor associated with permanent waves. Permanent wave odors are a great concern to hairstylists and clients. Many fear the odor is dangerous to their health, but odors themselves are not a danger. *In fact, odors can help you work more safely. Never judge a product's safety by its odor.*

An odor is caused by vapors touching the highly sensitive detectors in the nose. After the vapors leave the nose and enter the lungs, odor is no longer important. The lingering perm solution odor is from sulfur in the ATG. Hair and eggs both contain high amounts of sulfur, which is why perm odor is often described as smelling like rotten eggs.

Manufacturers often put fragrances into perms to help mask the odor. The reason is to remove some of the offensive smell, not to make the product safer. Simply removing or covering odors does not make the air any safer. Odors are no indication of a product's safety. In fact, odors can warn against overexposure.

Don't be fooled into believing that nicer smelling products are better or safer. The opposite is true, as well. Don't assume that foul smelling chemicals are dangerous to breathe. Permanent wave solutions are an excellent example. Perms smell foul, but the odor is not dangerous. Consult the MSDS to determine a product's potential hazards. Hazardous chemicals don't always smell unpleasant. Many are rather agreeable.

Of course, as previously discussed, always work with proper ventilation. Lowering inhalation exposure time is an important way to protect your health.

Many hairstylists take steps to avoid perm odors but fail to wear gloves or safety glasses. The real potential hazard for both alkaline and acid balance products is skin irritation and eye damage.

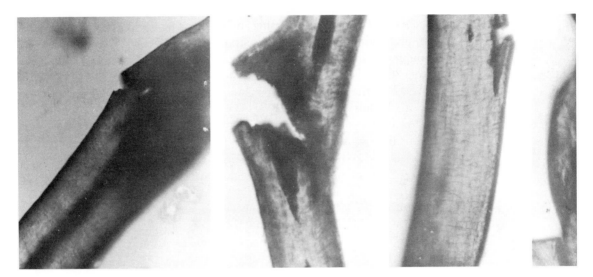

Figure 13-35 *Examples of hair damage caused by improper permanents.*
(*Courtesy: A. Langsam*)

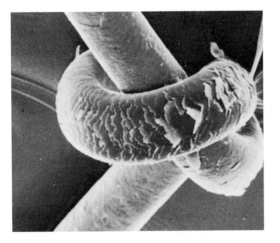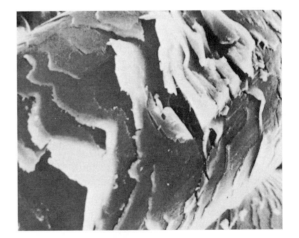

Figure 13-36 *Permanent-waved hair tied into a knot, shown at 630 times (left) and 1,600 times (right) magnification, emphasizes the cuticle damage caused by permanent waving.*
(*Courtesy: Gillette Company Research Institute, Rockville, Maryland*)

Scalp irritation (irritant contact dermatitis) may result from contact with the highly alkaline perm lotions.

Carefully examine the scalp and hair before beginning a perm procedure. Look for signs of scalp irritation, redness, tender or puffy tissue, open sores, excessive dryness, or other skin problems. If you spot a problem, advise the client to see a dermatologist before proceeding.

Alkaline substances are serious eye hazards. They may chemically react with eye protein and create a water-insoluble film. This film makes it difficult to flush the eye properly.

Permanent wave lotions and neutralizers are potentially dangerous to the eyes. Should eye contact occur, flush the eye immediately with warm, running water; then call a physician! Some chemicals have delayed effects and cause damage many hours later, if not properly treated.

To avoid accidents, wear proper eye protection. Use cotton bands to prevent products from dripping into the client's face. Clients expect you to protect their health.

Perm Problems

Hair is the fastest growing appendage of the human body. Anything that affects our general health also affects our hair. Diet, exercise, medications, and stress all affect the growth of our hair. The quality of any permanent wave corresponds to the quality of the hair. Strong hair usually produces strong curls, but weak hair usually produces weak curls.

Although it is sometimes suggested that factors such as menstrual cycle, pregnancy, surgeries, medication, etc., affect the final outcome of permanent waves, these beliefs have no scientific basis. The hair emerges from the scalp fully formed and keratinized. It is doubtful that hair that originated in the scalp years ago could be affected by one's menstrual cycle or pregnancy. No one has yet to prove a link between medications and permanent waving.

Permanent waving of hair involves science. More than likely, excuses for poor outcomes are simply that; excuses for doing a poor job.

Several factors for possible permanent wave failure are listed below:

1. Taking too large or too small a section

2. Using too much alkali product or improper mixing

3. Improper winding techniques or using the wrong rod size

4. Too short or long of a processing time

5. Failing to do a test curl

6. Improper rinsing and neutralizing

7. Incorrectly judging the hair's porosity, elasticity, and texture

8. Using the wrong product for the client's hair type

9. Not following manufacturer's directions

10. Not paying enough attention to directions and/or procedure

These reasons for perm failure make more sense than the excuses. If you patronize a fine restaurant and the food is terrible, would you blame the chef, or the ingredients? The same holds true for beauty salons. Clients come to the salon expecting professional results. They are looking for something better than they can do at home. Be sure you can provide the professional services clients are seeking.

REVIEW QUESTIONS

1. List and define the four major types of chemical bonds of the hair.
2. What part do reduction reactions play in permanent waves?
3. How do reducing agents and oxidizers work together to create a permanent wave?
4. Define hair shape and how it can be altered.
5. What are the major differences between alkaline and acid-balanced perms?
6. Explain why perm solutions have a strong characteristic odor.
7. Why are alkaline materials generally considered eye hazards?
8. Why is it important not to add additional alkaline material to perm lotions?
9. What could happen if perm lotion is not rinsed completely from the hair before neutralizing?
10. List all of the reasons why perms fail.

DISCUSSION QUESTIONS

1. What types of permanents contain potential sensitizers. How should hairstylists deal with this problem?
2. Discuss the action of reducing agents on the hair. How do they work?

Chapter 14

Chemical Hair Relaxers and Soft Curl Permanents

Key Terms

Base cream
Guanidine hydroxide relaxers
Hydroxide neutralizers
Hydroxide relaxers
Lanthionine bonds
Lanthionization
Lithium hydroxide and
　　potassium hydroxide
　　relaxers
Metal hydroxide relaxers
Sodium hydroxide relaxers
Soft curl permanents
Thio neutralizers
Thio relaxers

Learning Objectives

After completing this chapter, you should be able to:

- Understand the role that reduction reactions play in relaxers.

- Realize the importance of proper neutralization.

- Define lanthionization and how it relates to other chemical services.

- Effectively use prerelaxing evaluation tests to determine hair condition.

- Understand the difference between thio and hydroxide relaxers.

- Understand the difference between thio and hydroxide neutralizers.

CHEMICAL HAIR RELAXING

Chemical hair relaxing straightens overly curly hair. Permanent waving curls straight hair. Other than the objectives being so different, chemical hair relaxing is similar to permanent waving. The chemistry of thio relaxers and permanent waving is the same. Even though the chemistry of hydroxide relaxers and permanent waving is different, all relaxers and all permanents change the shape of the hair by breaking disulfide bonds.

These techniques require great care and attention. Errors may cause irreparable damage.

The concepts discussed in this chapter assume a basic understanding of hair structure and reduction/oxidation (redox) reactions.

A detailed guide to proper application and neutralization of relaxers is found in *Milady's Standard Textbook of Cosmetology*. This chapter will focus on the theory involved in those techniques.

HAIR RELAXING CHEMISTRY

Hair "remembers" its shape and will resist attempts to refashion it. Hair contains millions of disulfide cross-linked, polypeptide chains. The cross-link bonds work with peptide bonds, salt bonds, and hydrogen bonds to create amazingly strong structures. Curl removal is accomplished by breaking apart the cross-link side bonds.

Hair Types and Textures

A thorough understanding of the kind of hair to be straightened is necessary to minimize possible damage to the client's hair or scalp. It is important to detect the differences between the different types of hair and the action to be expected of the chemical hair relaxer.

Excessively Curly Hair

Excessively curly hair exists in all races. That means anyone of any race, or mixed race, can have excessively curly hair. It's also true that within races, individuals have hair with different degrees of curliness. African-Americans have hair of varying degrees of curliness, from nearly straight to excessively curly.

Excessively curly hair grows in long twisted spirals. Cross sections are highly elliptical and vary in shape and thickness along their length. Compared to straight or wavy hair, which tends to possess a fairly regular and uniform diameter along a single strand, excessively curly hair is fairly irregular, exhibiting varying diameters along a single strand.

The thinnest and weakest sections of the hair strand are located at the twists. These sections are also bent at a sharp angle and will be stretched the most during relaxing. A chain is only as strong as its weakest link and hair is only as strong as its weakest section. Hair breaks at its weakest point. Excessively curly hair usually breaks at the twists because of the weakness in that section and the extra physical force that is required to straighten it.

Fine Hair

The part of the hair that is to be straightened is the cortex. If the hair is fine and, therefore, has a smaller diameter than normal or average hair, the amount of cortex will be less. If the cuticle of the hair is not overly resistant, penetration of the relaxer will be quicker and processing time shorter.

Porous Hair

Porous hair, because of rather widely spaced cuticle scales, absorbs solutions more rapidly than normal hair and is naturally quicker to process. Less processing time should be allowed.

Coarse or Strong Hair

This type of hair usually has a larger diameter than normal hair and this results in a greater area of cortex. So more disulfide bonds need to be broken and processing time will be longer. If the cuticle is of the resistant type, processing time will be lengthened still more.

Dense Hair

This kind of hair thickly covers the scalp. As the follicles are numerous and closely clustered together, there are more hairs to be straightened. The hairstylist must use great care in applying sufficient amounts of chemical to ensure that all hairs are exposed equally to the relaxer.

Resistant Hair

This type of hair is less likely to be damaged by overprocessing with the relaxing chemical because the cuticle scales, being closer together, slow the rate of its penetration.

Sulfur Content

Some hair, usually red and black, has a higher sulfur content. This means that there are more disulfide bonds to be broken during the straightening process, lengthening the time required.

Prerelaxing Evaluations

Before relaxing the hair, three tests should be performed: an elasticity test, a strand test, and a porosity test. These tests, combined with careful observations allow the hairstylist to evaluate the hair's condition.

Elasticity is the hair's ability to withstand stretching or pulling. Normally, hair should have a great deal of elasticity. A loss of elasticity is a sign of damage. A strand of dry hair should stretch slightly without breaking.

To test for elasticity, stretch a single strand of dry hair between your fingers. Repeat this test in several locations. Hair that breaks under a slight strain has lost its elasticity. If the hair shows a large elasticity loss, examine it closely before proceeding. It requires special attention and several conditioning treatments before relaxing.

Strand testing gives warning of potential problems. Such tests show how the product works on the client's hair. Strand testing predicts what final results can be expected. Many factors affect the way hair responds to chemical treatments (e.g., porosity, texture, temperature, previous chemical services). Strand testing lessens the chance for unpleasant surprises. Proper testing takes these factors into account.

Apply the relaxer to a small section of hair, following the manufacturer's recommendations. If a section is more damaged, perform a second strand test on the damaged hair. Check the strands every three or four minutes until relaxation is complete. Rinse, neutralize, shampoo, and dry; then redo the elasticity test. Do not relax the hair if the test strands are very brittle or break easily.

To evaluate porosity properly, check different parts of the head, (i.e., the front hair line, behind the ear, and in the crown area). Gently slide a single strand of hair between your fingers, from the tip toward the scalp. Normal to resistant hair will feel smooth and silky. Roughness indicates a raised cuticle. Damaged hair will have a rough texture. Using a few dozen strands, repeat the test several times.

Each of these important tests helps evaluate the condition of the client's hair before relaxing. Prerelaxing evaluations are an important way to avoid overprocessing or causing excessive damage. They should be done before each service.

Overprocessing can be remedied with proper care and conditioning. However, hair in this condition cannot stand further damage. If these three tests indicate excessive hair damage, strongly encourage the client to delay the service. Suggest a conditioning program to correct the existing damage.

Thio Reduction Reactions

Thio relaxing solutions use reduction reactions to split disulfide bonds. While the relaxer cream is in contact with the cortex, the strong alkali softens and swells the hair. The thio breaks apart the disulfide bonds and the hair is in a *reduced state*.

The polypeptide chains of the cortex are unlinked by the bond breaking action of the chemical relaxer. This action will then permit the removal of excess curl from the hair. Bonds are rearranged into a straight position by *physical action*.

There are two forms of physical action—combing the chemical through the hair or using hands to pull the hair straight. Physically, the natural curl is removed by combing or pulling of the hair.

Gently pulling the hair with either a comb or hands shifts the broken disulfide bonds to new locations.

Caution: Hair in a reduced state is fragile and lacks strength. Be careful not to pull too hard. The peptide bonds can easily be broken. Rough handling can cause extensive hair damage.

There is a great similarity between the actions in permanent waving and in chemical hair straightening. In both cases, the disulfide bonds of the keratin are broken down in the softening process. In permanent waving, the hair is wound on rods in order that the softened hair will take the shape of the rod. The goal of permanent waving is to curl naturally straight hair.

In relaxing, the objective is the opposite. The goal is to straighten naturally curly hair. The disulfide bonds are shifted into a straight position by mechanical actions.

One of the differences between permanent waves and relaxers is the *viscosity* (thickness) of the chemical product. Relaxer products are thicker, having a much higher viscosity. Having a high viscosity in relaxers is an advantage. A thick product holds the hair in a straight position while it is being straightened/processed. Fatty materials and other hair conditioners are blended into a thickened cream base. This allows the relaxer to stay on the hair and not run off.

High viscosity would be a disadvantage in permanent waving lotions. The thickness would make application, rinsing, and neutralization difficult.

The two most common types of chemical hair relaxers are thio (ammonium thioglycolate or ATG) and hydroxide (OH^-) (see Appendix E).

Thio Relaxers

Caution: A thioglycolate relaxer product is incompatible with sodium hydroxide. Never use a thio relaxer on hair that has previously been relaxed with a sodium hydroxide product, or hair breakage may occur!

Thio (**THY**-oh) (ammonium thioglycolate or ATG) is the same reducing agent that is used in permanent waving. Other than the strength of the solution, their chemistry is identical. **Thio relaxers** may have a pH above 10 and a higher concentration of ATG than used in permanent waving. Thio relaxers are also thicker and have a higher viscosity.

Although the procedures are different, thio relaxers break disulfide bonds and soften hair, just like permanents (Chapter 13, Permanent Waving). After enough bonds are broken, the hair is straightened into its new shape and the relaxer is rinsed from the hair. Blotting comes next, followed by a neutralizer. The chemical reactions are identical to those in permanent waving.

Thio Neutralization

The **thio neutralizer** used with thio relaxers is an oxidizing agent, usually hydrogen peroxide, just like permanents. The oxidation reaction caused by the neutralizer rebuilds the disulfide bonds that were broken by the thio relaxer. The chemical reaction of the neutralizer is identical to the neutralizer used in permanent waving (Fig. 14–1 and Chapter 13, Permanent Waving).

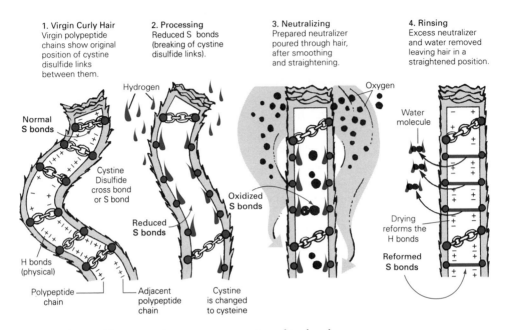

1. Virgin Curly Hair
Virgin polypeptide chains show original position of cystine disulfide links between them.

2. Processing
Reduced S bonds (breaking of cystine disulfide links).

3. Neutralizing
Prepared neutralizer poured through hair, after smoothing and straightening.

4. Rinsing
Excess neutralizer and water removed leaving hair in a straightened position.

Hydrogen

Oxygen

Water molecule

Normal S bonds

Cystine Disulfide cross bond or S bond

Reduced S bonds

Oxidized S bonds

Drying reforms the H bonds

Reformed S bonds

H bonds (physical)

Polypeptide chain

Adjacent polypeptide chain

Cystine is changed to cysteine

Figure 14-1 *Chemical hair straightening—ammonium thioglycolate.*

Soft Curl Permanents

A **soft curl permanent** is a combination of a thio relaxer, followed by a thio permanent wave that is wrapped on large rods. Soft curl permanents don't straighten the hair; they simply make the existing curl larger and looser. Soft curl permanents use ATG and oxidation neutralizers, just like thio permanent waves.

A soft curl permanent is actually two services. A soft curl permanent is a combination of a thio relaxer, followed by a thio permanent wave that is wrapped on large rods. Before excessively curly hair can be wrapped on rods (rodded), it must be relaxed with a thio relaxer. The process is the same as a thio relaxer, but the hair should not be neutralized before rodding. After the hair is relaxed it is wrapped on large rods and processed with a second thio solution. After processing, the hair is rinsed, blotted, and neutralized as with other permanents.

Hydroxide Relaxers (OH⁻)

There are several different types of hydroxide relaxers. The hydroxide ion (OH^-) is the active ingredient in all **hydroxide relaxers**. Sodium hydroxide, potassium hydroxide, lithium hydroxide, and guanidine hydroxide are all hydroxide relaxers. All hydroxide relaxers are strong alkalis (bases), which can swell the hair up to twice its normal diameter.

Hydroxide relaxers are not compatible with thio relaxers because they use a different chemistry. Thio relaxers have a pH of about 10 and use thio to break the disulfide bonds. The high pH of a thio relaxer simply opens the hair. Thio breaks the disulfide bonds.

Most hydroxide relaxers have an extremely high concentration of hydroxide ions (OH^-), which means they have a high pH (Chapter 9, Advanced Chemistry). The average pH of the hair is 5.0 and many hydroxide relaxers have a pH over 13.0. Since each step in the pH scale represents a tenfold change in concentration, a pH of 13.0 is one hundred million (100,000,000) times more alkaline than a pH of 5.0.

The hydroxide ion (OH^-) is the active ingredient in all hydroxide relaxers. The strength of all hydroxide relaxers is determined by the concentration of hydroxide ions, which is the pH of the relaxer. At high concentrations, the hydroxide ion breaks disulfide bonds by removing acidic hydrogen atoms next to the sulfur atoms in the disulfide bond. This is different than the reduction reaction caused by thio relaxers. The disulfide bonds that are broken by hydroxide relaxers are broken permanently and can never be reformed. Hydroxide relaxers work by a process called **lanthionization** (lan-thy-oh-ny-**ZAY**-shun). The disulfide bonds that are broken by hydroxide relaxers are converted to **lanthionine** (lan-**THY**-oh-neen) **bonds** when the relaxer is rinsed and the hair is still at a high pH (Fig. 14–2)

Thio Neutralization

Neutralization of a thio permanent or relaxer is an oxidation reaction that rebuilds the disulfide bonds that were broken during processing. Thio breaks disulfide bonds by adding extra hydrogen atoms to the two sulfur atoms joined in the disulfide bond. Neutralization, with an oxidizing agent, rebuilds the disulfide bonds by adding oxygen to the extra hydrogen atoms to form water. The formation of water removes the extra hydrogen atoms and allows the disulfide bonds to reform (Fig. 14–1 and Chapter 13, Permanent Waving).

Hydroxide Neutralization

Unlike permanent waving neutralization, the neutralization of hydroxide relaxers does not involve an oxidation reaction. Hydroxide neutralizers neutralize the alkaline residues (OH^-) left in the hair by the relaxer. The pH of hydroxide relaxers is so high that the hair remains at a high pH, even after thorough rinsing. Since acids neutralize alkalis (Chapter 9, Advanced Chemistry), the application of an acid-balanced shampoo or a normalizing lotion neutralizes any remaining hydroxide ions and lowers the pH of the hair and scalp. Some neutralizing shampoos, intended for use after hydroxide relaxers, have pH indicators that will change color to indicate if the pH of the hair has returned to normal.

Since the disulfide bonds that have been broken by hydroxide relaxers cannot be reformed by oxidation, application of a neutralizer that contains an

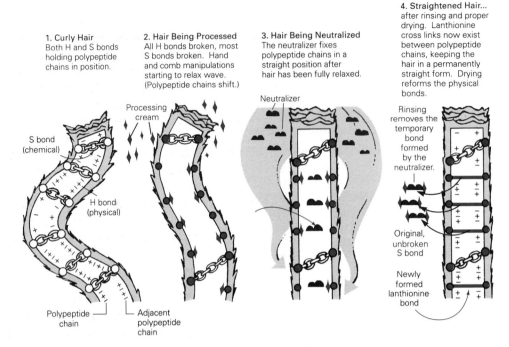

Figure 14-2 *Chemical hair straightening — sodium hydroxide.*

oxidizing agent will not rebuild the disulfide bonds and will only damage the hair. Disulfide bonds that have been broken by hydroxide relaxers cannot be reformed.

Hair that has been treated with hydroxide relaxers is unfit for thio relaxers or permanent waving. Disulfide bonds that are broken by hydroxide relaxers are converted to lanthionine bonds (Fig. 14–2). Unlike disulfide bonds, which are formed with two sulfur atoms, lanthionine bonds are formed with a single sulfur atom. Thio relaxers and thio permanents are designed to break disulfide bonds, not lanthionine bonds. The application of a thio relaxer or thio permanent on hair that has been treated with a hydroxide relaxer will not properly relax, or curl, the hair and may cause extreme damage. **Hair that has been treated with hydroxide relaxers is unfit for thio relaxers or permanent waving.**

Metal Hydroxide Relaxers

Metal hydroxide relaxers are ionic compounds formed by a metal, sodium (Na), potassium (K), or lithium (Li), which is combined with oxygen (O) and hydrogen (H). Metal hydroxide relaxers include sodium hydroxide (NaOH), potassium hydroxide (KOH), and lithium hydroxide (LiOH).

All metal hydroxide relaxers contain only one component and are used, without mixing, exactly as they are packaged in the container. The hydroxide ion (OH⁻) is the active ingredient in all hydroxide relaxers. There is no significant difference in the straightening ability of these metal hydroxide relaxers.

Sodium Hydroxide

Caution: A sodium hydroxide relaxer is incompatible with thioglycolate. Never use a sodium hydroxide product on hair that has been previously relaxed with a thioglycolate product, or hair breakage may occur!

Sodium hydroxide is commonly used in chemical relaxing products and is an effective hair straightener. Sodium hydroxide is also known as lye or caustic soda. The pH level of this product often exceeds 13 and is sometimes above 13.5! As this high pH level suggests, this is a highly corrosive chemical. The hair can swell to more than twice its normal diameter. Use this relaxer with care and caution.

Sodium hydroxide is the same chemical used in drain cleaners and chemical hair depilatories.

Lithium Hydroxide and Potassium Hydroxide

Lithium hydroxide (LiOH) and **potassium hydroxide** (KOH) are sometimes advertised and sold as "no mix–no lye" relaxers. Although, technically, they are not lye, the chemistry is identical, with little difference in their performance. The hydroxide ion (OH⁻) is the active ingredient in all hydroxide relaxers. All metal hydroxide relaxers share the same chemistry, which makes them incompatible with thio permanents and relaxers.

Guanidine Hydroxide

Guanidine (GWAN-ih-deen) **hydroxide relaxers** are usually advertised and sold as "no lye" relaxers. Although, technically, they are not lye, the hydroxide ion (OH⁻) is still the active ingredient. Guanidine hydroxide relaxers have the same basic chemistry as all other hydroxide relaxers, which make them incompatible with all thio permanents and relaxers.

Guanidine hydroxide relaxers contain two components that must be mixed immediately prior to use. Mixing a cream, containing calcium hydroxide, with a liquid activator, containing guanidine carbonate, causes a chemical reaction that produces guanidine hydroxide. Calcium hydroxide and guanidine carbonate will not straighten hair unless they are mixed correctly and in the exact proportions. Even though calcium hydroxide is often found in depilatories or added to metal hydroxide relaxers, calcium hydroxide, alone, will not straighten hair.

Guanidine hydroxide relaxers have the ability to straighten hair completely with significantly less scalp irritation than other hydroxide relaxers. Most guanidine hydroxide relaxers are recommended for sensitive scalp and sold over the counter for home use. Although guanidine hydroxide relaxers reduce scalp irritation, they don't reduce hair damage. Guanidine hydroxide relaxers swell the hair slightly more than other hydroxide relaxers and are also more drying, especially after repeated applications.

Base and No-base Formulas

Hydroxide relaxers are usually sold in base and no-base formulas. **Base cream** is a petroleum cream that is applied to the skin and scalp to provide a barrier designed to protect the client's skin from irritation. For added protection, *base formulas* require the application of base cream to the entire scalp, prior to the application of the relaxer.

No-base relaxers already contain a base cream in the oil phase of the emulsion that is designed to melt at body temperature. As the relaxer is applied, body heat causes the base to melt and settle out on the scalp, in a thin, oily, protective coating. As added protection, base cream should always be applied to the entire hairline and around the ears, even with no-base relaxers.

Low pH Relaxers

Some reducing agents work fairly well at pH levels between 6.5 and 8.5. Sodium bisulfite is an example of a low pH value reducing agent. Low pH relaxers are less effective in straightening hair, especially resistant hair. However, they are milder on the scalp and hair. These relaxers are recommended for thin or overly brittle hair.

Use these relaxing agents with great care and caution. If used incorrectly, they cause serious scalp and skin burns. These same chemicals are used in depilatory creams and can dissolve hair.

These chemicals are highly corrosive to the skin and eyes. Always wear safety glasses and gloves when mixing, measuring, pouring, or dispensing the substances. Take precautions to protect clients, as well.

As discussed in previous chapters, the rate of a chemical reaction doubles with each 18°F/10°C rise in temperature. Therefore, using heat to speed up the relaxing process can be dangerous. The corrosive action on skin will speed up, as well. Never use heat unless specified in the manufacturer's instructions.

Use extreme caution with all types of relaxers. Always keep these products from contacting a client's skin, i.e., ears, forehead, and neck. Applying protective cream to these areas is advisable even with no-base products.

Relaxer Timing

Improper timing of hair relaxing services is a common and potentially serious error. This can be dangerous to the client. It is important to develop a foolproof system for timing hair relaxing services.

Always use a timer with an alarm. Check the client's hair periodically. This improves the quality of service and helps avoid overprocessing. Used improperly, relaxers with extremely high pH levels can rapidly destroy hair and skin.

Although they frequently occur, problems of this nature are unnecessary. Relaxers have been used safely for many years by thousands of clients. With care and attention, clients should never experience problems.

HAIR RELAXING SAFETY

Scalp irritation (irritant contact dermatitis) sometimes results from relaxer products. Shampooing before the relaxing service will increase the risk of irritation. The scalp has a protective barrier of sebum that is temporarily removed by shampooing.

Ask clients to refrain from shampooing their hair for twenty-four hours prior to a chemical relaxer application. You may wish to recommend the client use a buildup-removing shampoo for several shampoos before the appointment. Never shampoo a client's hair before applying a chemical relaxer. This is especially important for hydroxide relaxers.

Examine the scalp and hair carefully before beginning a chemical relaxer treatment. Look for signs of scalp irritation, redness, tender or puffy tissue, open sores, and excessive dryness or other skin problems. If a problem is observed, advise the client to see a dermatologist before proceeding with a chemical service.

In general, high-alkaline products are serious eye hazards. They may chemically react with eye protein and create a water-insoluble film. This film makes it difficult to flush and cleanse the eye properly.

Relaxers and neutralizers are potentially dangerous to the eyes. Should accidental contact occur, flush the eye immediately with warm, running water. Then call a physician! Some chemicals have delayed effects, causing damage hours later if not properly treated.

To avoid accidents, wear proper eye protection. Use protective creams to prevent contact with the client's face, ears, or neck.

A common mistake is made when retouching regrowth. Use every precaution to avoid overlapping. Overlapping previously relaxed hair can lead to hair breakage and excessive damage.

Proper shampooing and rinsing is an important final step. Relaxer residues are trapped beneath the cuticle layer. Failing to neutralize residues completely causes excessive and continuing damage.

Follow the manufacturer's directions when rinsing and neutralizing. After neutralizing, flush with an acid rinse, then shampoo with a mild, acid shampoo and apply a conditioner. Take care to massage the scalp gently. This prevents further irritation to sensitive tissue (Figs. 14–3 thru 14–9).

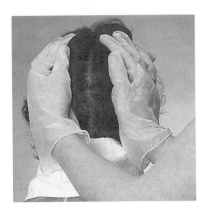

Figure 14-3 *Examining the scalp.*

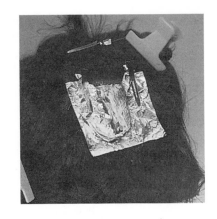

Figure 14-4 *Relaxer strand test.*

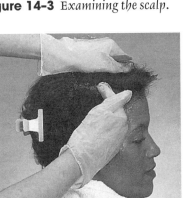

Figure 14-5 *Applying protective base.*

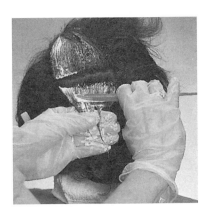

Figure 14-6 *Applying relaxer on top of strand.*

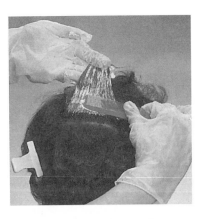

Figure 14-7 *Applying relaxer underneath strand.*

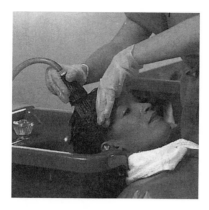

Figure 14-8 *Rinsing out relaxer.*

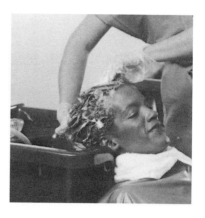

Figure 14-9 *Shampooing the hair.*

REVIEW QUESTIONS

1. List the difference between permanent waving lotions and relaxers made with ammonium thioglycolate.
2. Why is hair in the reduced state more fragile?
3. How do thio neutralizers work?
4. What chemicals are used to dissolve hair?
5. Why do some relaxers use a base cream?
6. What is the difference between lanthionine and disulfide bonds?
7. In what three ways should hair be evaluated before relaxing the hair?
8. List safety procedures and precautions to be observed while using relaxers.

DISCUSSION QUESTIONS

1. A client comes to you after doing a "home" permanent wave with poor results. The client wants the curls relaxed but the hair was severely over-processed by the perm lotion. You perform a strand test and an elasticity

test, and check the porosity. The results tell you the client's hair might not stand the process, but the client insists.

Discuss the various alternatives. For example:

a. You refuse and advise a hair-conditioning program.

b. You perform the service and badly burn the hair.

c. Can you think of other possibilities?

Chapter 15

Salon Health and Safety

Learning Objectives

After completing this chapter, you should be able to:

- Understand the importance of working safely.

- Explain how chemicals affect our every day lives.

- Explain how the "overexposure principle" can protect you.

- List the rules of working safely.

- Understand the importance of Material Safety Data Sheets (MSDSs).

- Choose and use the proper safety equipment.

- Define toxicity and carcinogenicity.

- Protect your health while working in the salon.

Take the time to learn the rules of working safely with salon chemicals. Why risk the consequences? In the salon, achieving superior results for clients is the ultimate goal, but don't stop there. Keep clients happy and keep your body healthy too! Both of these goals require knowledge and careful attention to safety.

Learn to use products correctly and safely. Study the manufacturer's educational literature and read the warning labels. Always handle, mix, and store products following directions of the experts. The experts include the manufacturer and federal and state agencies that monitor product research, use, and disposal. Use products in strict accordance with the manufacturer's instructions and follow the rules of working safely. Remember safety and health come first!

THE IMPORTANCE OF WORKING SAFELY

What is a chemical? In chapter 8, we learned that everything you can see and touch is a chemical, except for light and electricity. Air is a combination of many chemicals (i.e., oxygen, hydrogen, and nitrogen). Clean, pure mountain stream water is a chemical. Hair is long polypeptide chains of chemicals.

Many people believe that all chemicals are dangerous or toxic substances. Ask your friends what they think of when they hear the word *chemicals*. Toxic waste dumps or factories dumping poisonous waste into streams?

People fear chemicals because they have little understanding of chemistry. The news media often use the word *chemical* in a scary, negative way.

Understanding chemical tools will help put you in control and help clients understand products. Working safely is very easy to do, if you know how and read and follow directions. However, irresponsible or careless use may result in serious accidents or permanent damage to you or a client's health.

THE RULES OF WORKING SAFELY

FACT #1: Most chemicals are not harmful unless you overexpose yourself to the substance.

Is it possible to work safely with potentially dangerous chemicals? Of course it is if you read the literature. Safety doesn't just happen. You must learn the facts and obey the rules of working safely.

All hairstylists should learn and remember the *overexposure principle*. This rule says, "Every chemical substance used in a salon has a safe and unsafe level of exposure. Simply coming in contact with a potentially hazardous substance should not cause you harm. The danger is exceeding the safe level of exposure."

Chemicals that are identified as dangerous at low levels are not suitable for use in the salon. Profession products are formulated to be as safe as possible. Still, no cosmetic chemical is completely free from risks.

You are ultimately responsible for proper use and safe handling of the chemicals. A normally safe product can become dangerous if used incorrectly. Workers in all professions must follow safe working procedures.

How can this be done? Product knowledge, proper training in chemical use, and information are the key factors.

RULE #1: Look for ways to reduce chemical exposure to safe levels.

The **Occupational Safety and Health Administration (OSHA)** is responsible for enforcing a federal law designed to help you work smartly and safely. This agency includes regulations for the *Hazard Communication Standard* or the *Employee Right to Know Act*. Employees who work with chemicals on the job are affected by OSHA regulations. They include the following:

1. Information about hazardous ingredients must be provided to all employees.

2. Employers must train employees to understand this information properly.

3. Employers are required to provide a safe working environment.

When children are shown how to pick up broken glass safely without getting cut, they are learning to perform a potentially dangerous task without being harmed. That's what working safely is all about! Even simple tasks become dangerous when done incorrectly.

The Hazard Communication Standard requires manufacturers to specify information about a product's safety. This vital information is found on special forms called **Material Safety Data Sheets (MSDSs).** (Appendix E) Your local distributors of beauty supplies must supply you with MSDSs for the products that you buy from them. You are responsible for collecting these sheets and keeping them available for reference. If you have difficulty collecting the MSDSs you need, send a formal written request to the distributor.

MSDSs provide information to many types of workers who handle chemicals; MSDSs help firefighters deal with chemical fires and clean up chemical spills. Information on an MSDS often helps doctors treat accidental poisonings.

Understanding MSDSs is as important as learning proper application techniques.

Here is a brief list of what is shown on an MSDS:

- Potentially hazardous ingredients found in each product
- Properly store and safely use chemical products
- Ways to prevent hazardous chemicals from entering the body
- The short-term and long-term health effects of overexposure
- Early warning signs of product overexposure
- Emergency first-aid advice
- Safe handling techniques

The MSDSs teach you how to work safely and avoid risks (Fig 15–1). Knowing that a chemical may cause a blood disorder isn't as important as avoiding exposure that can cause a blood disorder. Working safely is an important part of the

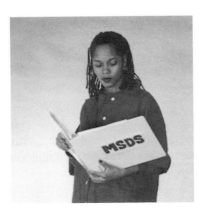

Figure 15-1 *Read your* MSDSs.

hairstylist's profession. Being a professional means more than creating beautiful hair. Professionals must work responsibly with trade tools and products. This is what sets a professional apart from the nonprofessional.

Proper Storage Conditions

Improper storage of chemicals can create many problems. Improper storage may ruin a product or shorten its shelf life. It can also cause a fire or explosion. Extreme cold, excessive heat, and light adversely affect many products.

Flammable products must be stored away from heat or any source of flame (e.g., away from cigarettes, heaters, window sills). Never carry any product in a car trunk. Many salon chemicals are as flammable as gasoline.

Chemicals should always be kept in their original, marked containers. For maximum stability and safety, always store chemicals in a cool, dry location away from sunlight and excessive heat or cold.

Hydrogen peroxide (H_2O_2) demonstrates the importance of proper storage. Storing (H_2O_2) in sealed, metal containers can cause violent explosions.

The information on the MSDS also helps you avoid other dangerous conditions, such as dangerous mixtures that might emit toxic fumes or cause fires.

Keeping Salon Chemicals Out of Your Body

Chemicals can enter your body by three routes:

1. Inhalation of vapors, mists, or dusts

2. Absorption through the skin or broken tissue

3. Unintentional or accidental ingestion

The information on the MSDSs warn you of the possible *route of entry* for each product. Lowering chemical exposure is easier if you know which products are dangerous to breathe and which should not come in contact with the skin.

Health Effects

The MSDSs explain both short-term and long-term effects of overexposure. Short-term effects (**acute effects**) result from overexposure for short periods. Typically, working 40 hours a week for three months or less is considered short term.

Long-term effects (**chronic effects**) can occur with overexposure or misuse. Adverse health effects often begin after several years of repeated overexposure.

The information on the MSDSs might not list any negative health effects, but don't assume that the product cannot cause you harm. Handle salon chemicals with respect and follow the instructions. Be extra careful when mixing products. Mixing some products together can cause unwanted and dangerous chemical reactions. The most common example is mixing chlorine bleach with ammonia or an acid. Chlorine bleach will react with ammonia or an acid to form deadly chlorine gas. Exposure to chlorine gas can be fatal after just a few minutes of exposure in a poorly ventilated area.

Make sure you carefully read the labels on products before mixing. For example, mixing the activator tube from an acid-balanced permanent with the neutralizer, instead of the waving solution, can cause a violent explosion. The activator tube in acid waves contains glyceryl monothioglycolate (GMTG), which is added to the waving solution immediately prior to use (Chapter 13, Permanent Waving). Neutralizers are oxidizing agents, usually peroxide. Adding the activator (thioglycolate) to the neutralizer (peroxide), by mistake, will result in a violent, explosive, exothermic oxidation reaction.

> **FACT #2:** Scientists are constantly learning about the dangerous properties of chemicals.

The reaction involved in this accident is the same reaction that takes place in exothermic waves. The only difference is in the concentration of reactants and the rate of reaction. The activator in exothermic permanents contains hydrogen peroxide. When the activator (peroxide) is added to the permanent waving solution (thioglycolate) an exothermic oxidation reaction takes place, which causes the solution to heat up. The rate of this reaction is slow due to the small concentration of peroxide in the activator, far less than the concentration of peroxide in the neutralizer. As in most chemical reactions, increasing the concentration of reactants increases the amount and rate of reaction.

> **RULE #2:** The products you use are tools, not toys! Treat them with respect.

Oxidizers that are mixed with alkaline chemicals or placed in metal containers will expand and get hot. Hydrogen peroxide that has been contaminated, or is stored in the wrong container, can heat up and explode.

Remember, adverse health effects are not likely to happen if you use products correctly. However, problems might arise if you misuse or abuse the product.

Always work safely and follow directions precisely.

Signs and Symptoms of Overexposure

The human body is wonderfully complex. The body will often give early warning signs when chemical products are not being used safely. Different chemicals cause different early warning signs.

For example, overexposure to some solvents can make you feel very tired or may keep you from sleeping. Overexposure to other chemicals can cause headaches, nausea, angry or frustrated feelings, nosebleeds, tingling fingers and toes, dry or scratchy nose and throat, puffy red and irritated skin, itching, and many other symptoms.

Understanding and watching for unusual symptoms helps hairstylists avoid more serious, long-term problems. Pay attention to how your body reacts.

Emergency and First Aid Treatment

FACT #3: Accidents usually occur when they are least expected.

RULE #3: Be prepared! Read, learn, and get some training! Plan ahead for accidents.

If a serious accident happens in a salon, what do you do? Only after the fact do people often discover that they are unprepared to treat or respond to accidents.

The MSDS may help provide answers to these questions during a time of crisis.

Our next rule is a familiar one.

What should you do if a small child, running through the salon, grabs a bottle of permanent wave solution and drinks some of it? By the time you remember where you put the phone number to the poison control center, it could be too late. Plan ahead; you may save a life (Fig. 15–2).

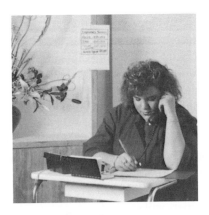

Figure 15-2 *Be prepared to handle accidents. Don't wait until after an accident has happened to figure out how to handle it. Have the poison control number and other emergency numbers near the phone.*

Safe Handling Techniques

Each job requires different tools and techniques. The same is true when using professional salon chemicals. Each chemical requires different handling for safe use.

For example, quickly evaporating solvents require appropriate ventilation during use to remove vapors. Safety glasses should be worn to prevent chemicals from splashing in the eyes. Other products may require a special type of glove or extra precautions to prevent fires.

The manufacturer's instructions and the information on the MSDSs will help guide you. If either of these suggests that you wear safety glasses, it is for good reason. Manufacturers are the voice of experience. Use this information to your advantage. It is your responsibility.

You can find useful information on the MSDS. Become accustomed to reading MSDSs. Properly using these important resources is wise. The world of hairstyling is constantly changing. Keeping pace with the industry means keeping up with the changes. Don't let your education end when you leave school; continue with lifelong learning.

Using and Choosing Safety Equipment

Actually, working safely is surprisingly easy! Still, each year some hairstylists suffer needless harm or injury. Following rules of safety will help protect you from hazards in the salon.

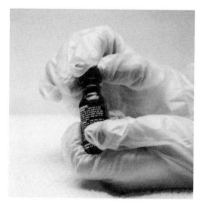

Figure 15–3 *Wear gloves whenever recommended by the manufacturer's instructions or MSDS.*

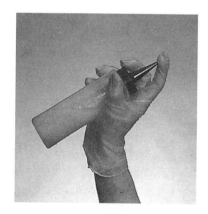

Figure 15–4 *Wear gloves when preparing and mixing formulas.*

Remember that chemicals enter the body through three routes of entry:

- **Inhalation** of vapors, mists, and dusts
- **Absorption** through the skin or broken tissue
- Accidental or unintentional **ingestion**

Blocking these routes helps lower your exposure to safe levels.

Volatile solvents are those which evaporate quickly. Some liquids evaporate slowly but still form vapors. What is the best and easiest way to avoid inhaling excessive amounts of harmful **vapors**? Use techniques (good ventilation) that keep vapors from getting into the air you breathe.

Closing product containers reduces the amount of vapor released into the air. Besides, it helps keep products fresh and effective. An open container can be an accident waiting to happen.

Quickly wipe up spills, especially chemicals. Using waste cans with covers to help keep vapors out of the air is recommended.

Mists are actually tiny liquid droplets that rapidly evaporate into the air. Spraying any chemical into the air increases the risk of excessive inhaling and overexposure. For example, pressurized aerosol containers produce fine and lingering mists. A fine mist is difficult to control and usually more hazardous to breathe. Pump sprayers create larger droplets that are less hazardous. Avoid spraying excessive amounts of products into the air.

Surgical-type dust masks are ineffective against vapors. These masks should only be used to keep dust particles out of your lungs. Some high-quality masks are also effective against mists (i.e., hair sprays). The instructions that come with the masks tell you whether they can be used for both dust and mist. Also, throw away dust masks daily; they quickly lose effectiveness.

Using products that cover up or remove odors from the salon will not protect people against health hazards. Simply removing odors will not make the air safer to breathe. Odors are no indication of product safety; however, odors can warn against overexposure. An odor is nothing more than vapors touching the highly sensitive detectors in the nose. After the vapors leave the nose and enter the lungs, the odor is no longer important.

You are asking for trouble if you use an odor to judge product safety. Hazardous chemicals don't always smell unpleasant. Many are rather agreeable and pleasant to smell.

Proper ventilation removes vapors from the room and expels them from the building. Any system designed to clean the air will not be as effective.

Working Smart

Question: What do a coffee cup, a piece of chocolate, and a sack lunch have in common?

Give up? These are all ways that hairstylists EAT their chemical products. Sadly, hairstylists eat far more product than they realize.

FACT #4: All liquids evaporate and form vapors.

RULE #4: Keep products capped or covered when not in use. Also, empty waste containers regularly (at least three times a day).

FACT #5: A vapor molecule is hundreds of times smaller than a dust particle.

RULE #5: Never use a dust mask to protect yourself from vapors. Vapors are far too small to be filtered by dust masks.

FACT #6: Odors themselves are not dangerous. In fact, odors can help you work more safely.

RULE #6: Never judge product safety by odor.

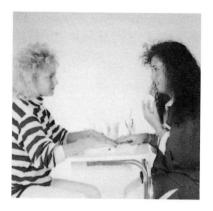

Figure 15-5 *Never eat or drink in the salon area. You will be eating or drinking your products.*

- Coffee cups can easily collect dusts and powders. Hot liquids like coffee and tea will also absorb vapors right out of the air.
- When someone offers you a piece of chocolate or you dodge into the kitchen for a cookie, do you always think to wash your hands first?

Accidental product ingestion is easy to do in the salon. Watch for young children, too. They are curious and may grab open bottles.

Protect Your Eyes

Accidents involving the eyes are a serious danger in salons. Solvents in the eye can be very painful and may cause severe damage. Hydrogen peroxide, permanent wave solutions, and neutralizers are just a few of the chemicals that may cause eye injury or blindness.

Wear eye protection whenever there is the slightest chance that a chemical product may get into your eyes. Eye injuries account for approximately 45 percent of the cosmetic-related injuries seen in hospital emergency rooms.

Seldom do salons lose business because hairstylists worked safely or showed concern for a customer's well-being (Figs. 15–6 through 15–8).

Wearing contact lenses in the salon is risky. Vapors collect on the soft contact lenses and make them unwearable. The contaminated lens may etch the surface of the eye. Should an accidental splash get into the eye, contact lenses hinder proper natural cleaning of the eye. The contact lenses should be removed and the eye properly flushed should a splash of liquid get into the eye.

Most of these rules are common sense. When using salon chemicals, applying common sense may save you from pain and suffering. Learn the chemical safety rules and practice them!

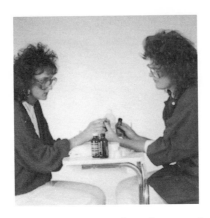

Figure 15-6 *Wear safety glasses and give your client a pair.*

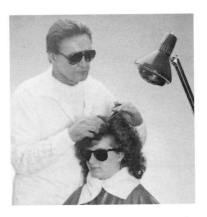

Figure 15-7 *Protect your eyes and your client's eyes during a scalp treatment.*

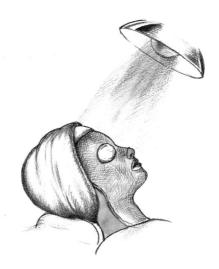

Figure 15-8 *Protect your client's eyes during a facial treatment.*

FACT #10: A chemical is considered to be relatively nontoxic only if drinking a quart or more won't cause death.

RULE #10: Treat all chemical products with respect. Don't be fooled by marketing terms like *nontoxic, natural,* and *organic*.

TOXICITY AND CARCINOGENICITY

Toxic substances are usually thought of as being dangerous poisons. The news media use the term *toxic* often and the general public fears its very mention. Should hairstylists avoid any product that is toxic? The answer to this question will surprise you.

Paracelsus, a famous 14th-century physician, was the first to use the word "toxic." He said, "All substances are poisons; there is none which is not a poison. The right dose differentiates a poison and a remedy." Over the last 500 years, the public has forgotten what Paracelsus discovered. The overexposure principle is the modern-day interpretation of Paracelsus's discovery. If you remember, this principle also says that the dose level (overexposure) determines toxicity.

Next time someone tells you a product is nontoxic, think about this definition. This type of claim is actually deceptive.

Remember your chemistry? Organic simply means that the chemical contains carbon in its structure. Rat poison and road tar are both organic!

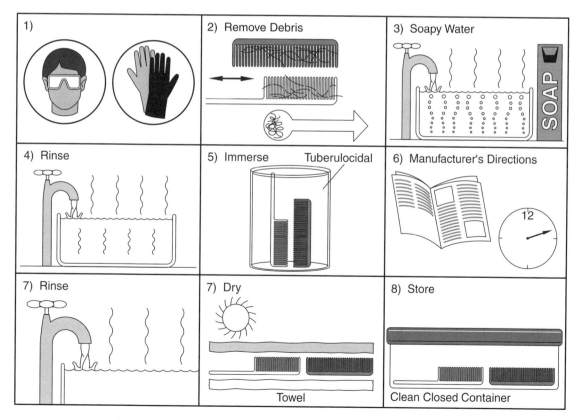

Figure 15-9 *Step by step procedure for decontaminating implements.*

Carcinogenicity

The media have treated the topic of **carcinogenic** (cancer-causing) chemicals in an irresponsible manner. According to the news, nearly everything causes cancer, right? WRONG!

Don't let these exaggerated reports frighten you. If you work safely, product exposure or use will probably not cause cancer. The cancer risks from cigarettes are hundreds (maybe thousands) of times greater. Besides, even chemicals that may cause serious illnesses, can only cause harm if you overexpose yourself for a prolonged period.

Overexposure to many salon chemicals can cause illness, but overexposure is unnecessary and risky. These useful substances can be used safely, without posing a health risk.

Ultimately, you are responsible for preventing accidents and protecting your health! Learn what you can about working safely and obey the rules. You may become the best hairstylist in the state, but it won't mean anything if you harm yourself in the process. Don't just talk about working safely, it only works if you really do it!

RULES OF SAFETY

1. Look for ways to reduce chemical exposure to safe levels.

2. The products you use are tools, not toys! Treat them with respect.

3. Be prepared! Read, learn, and get some training! Plan ahead for accidents

4. Keep products capped or covered when not in use. Also, empty waste containers regularly (at least daily).

5. Never use a dust mask to protect yourself from vapors. Vapors are far too small to be filtered by dust masks.

6. Never judge product safety by odor.

7. Never eat or drink in the salon. Always store food away from salon chemicals and wash your hands before eating.

8. Wear approved safety glasses whenever you work.

9. It is not advisable to wear contact lenses in the salon and always wash your hands before touching the eye area.

10. Treat all chemical products with respect. Don't be fooled by marketing terms like nontoxic, natural, and organic.

11. Don't judge a chemical by what it CAN do. What's important is how easily you can prevent any potential hazard.

REVIEW QUESTOINS

1. Write a paragraph (use your own words) that explains both the Overexposure Principle and Paracelsus's philosophy.

2. List seven important pieces of information found on an MSDS.

3. Name the routes of entry and give examples of a safety technique that can block each route.

4. What is the "best" way to help keep salon air free from hazardous chemical vapors?

5. Against which kind of salon hazard are surgical type masks most effective? Against which salon hazard are they ineffective?

6. Name five symptoms of chemical overexposure.

7. To work safely with chemicals you must lower your _____ to _____ levels.

8. List three ways that accidental ingestion of salon products might occur.

9. What percentage of salon chemicals can never be toxic under any circumstances?

DISCUSSION QUESTIONS

1. List the steps that you can take to protect yourself from overexposure.

2. Make an emergency action plan that lists the proper steps to take in the event of an emergency.

Conclusion

The most beautiful thing we can experience is the mysterious. It is the true source of art and science.

Albert Einstein

It seems appropriate to repeat this quote from the first chapter.

No profession on earth blends art and science more beautifully than hairstyling. However, there is no mystery about what makes a hairstylist a true professional. The technological revolution propelled the industry into a new era. The rapid scientific advancements of the last decade present hairstylists with new priorities and challenges. To keep pace, you must continue to learn and improve your knowledge.

Challenge your imagination to find uses for this knowledge and your success will be limited only by your imagination.

Appendix A | Safety Information

Lab Safety Supply
P.O. Box 1368
Janesville, WI 53547-1368
(800) 356-0783
www.Labsafety.com

This company sells primarily to the chemical industry, but is an excellent source of safety equipment ranging from gloves and eye protection to masks and ventilation. Its *Fume Vac* and *Fume Extractor* are no-hype, first-rate salon ventilation systems. They also offer a Safety Techline (800) 356-2501, which can be very useful in deciding which equipment is right for you.

Occupational Safety and Health Administration (OSHA)
U.S. Department of Labor
Technical Data Center
Washington, D.C. 20210
(202) 693-1888
www.osha.gov

OSHA provides information concerning regulations and job safety. It is also responsible for enforcing the Hazard Communication Standard (Employee Right to Know Act). Also, check with your county seat or state capital for local and district offices near you.

Hazard Evaluation System & Information Service
California Occupational Health Program
2151 Berkeley Way
Berkeley, CA 94704
(510) 540-3138

This organization has written an excellent, free booklet which explains the hazards of many common chemicals. A must for anyone working in the salon industry. Order by mail or call the number listed.

FDA Cosmetics Technology Division
Food and Drug Administration
5600 Fisher Lane
Rockville, MD 20857
(202) 205-4706

(202) 401-2242
http//:vm.cfsan.fds.gov

Contrary to popular belief, the FDA does not test cosmetic products, and does not insure the safety of cosmetics. Manufacturers are solely responsible for the safety of their product line.

Should you experience a serious, cosmetic-related problem that cannot be resolved with the manufacturer, write to the FDA. Unless the FDA hears about serious problems, it can do nothing.

The FDA is not a cosmetic-approving organization; that's your job! The FDA is a cosmetic-disapproving organization. It is a useful and necessary part of the effort to improve the safety and quality of cosmetics ingredients.

Appendix B | Common Irritants and Allergens

Contact Irritants

Soaps, detergents, and shampoo
Permanent wave lotions (all pH levels)
Bleaches
Water
Ammonium thioglycolate
Peroxides (all types)
Oxidizers and neutralizers
Ammonia

Contact Allergens

Lanolin (skin and hair care)
p-Phenylenediamine (haircolor)
Rubber glove additives
Nickel (nickel sulfate from tools, i.e., shears)
Rosin (depilatories)
Balsam of Peru (conditioners)
Captan (preservative, antidandruff ingredient)
DMDM hydantion (skin care ingredient)
Glyceryl monothioglycolate (low pH level permanent-wave lotion)
Hydroquinone (bleaches)
Lavender oil
Essential oil concentrates (Many natural oils are strong irritants.)
Propylene glycol
Ammonium persulfate (bleach booster)
Imidazolidinyl urea (preservative)
Quanternium 15 (preservative)
Formaldehyde (preservative, nail hardener)
Benzalkonium chloride (germicide)
BHA (preservative, antioxidant)
Methyl and/or propyl paraben (preservatives)
Many types of fragrances (both natural and synthetic)

Appendix C | Patch Testing Directions

1. The hair dye in this package must never be used for dyeing hair unless a preliminary skin test has been made. The skin test must be made each and every time before the hair is to be dyed, regardless of whether or not a skin test has been made at some time previously.

2. The dye used for the preliminary test must be a portion of the article intended to be used for dyeing the hair.

3. The sample of dye to be used for preliminary skin test should be mixed and prepared in exactly the same manner and according to the directions applicable to the actual use of the hair dye itself.

4. By means of a suitable applicator (clean camel's hair brush, cotton-tipped applicator, or other applicator), a streak of dye not less than a quarter of an inch wide and at least one-half inch long is made on the skin and scalp behind one ear. It is important that the streak of dye extend into the hair portions of the scalp as well as that portion of the skin that is hairless.

5. The streak of dye should be permitted to remain for at least twenty-four hours. The test should be read between twenty-four and forty-eight hours after application. Preferably the text area should not be covered with any type of dressing and contact with comb, hats, spectacles or any other objects should be avoided.

6. Warning: If redness, burning, itching, small blisters, or any type of eruption appears in the general area used for the skin test during the first twenty-four hours, the individual is sensitive to the dye, and under no circumstances should it be used for dyeing the hair. Hair dyes should not be used when there is any disease or eruption present anywhere on the skin or on the scalp.

Appendix D | Science, Lab Equipment, and Industry Resources

Edmund Scientific Company
Consumer Science Division
101 East Gloucester Pike
Barrington, NJ 08007-1380
(800) 728-6999
www.scientificsonline.com

Microscopes, optics, biology, posters, chemicals, and assorted science projects and teaching aids.

Nasco
4825 Stoddard Road
Modesto, CA 95356-9318
(800) 558-9595 or (209) 545-1600

Chemicals, laboratory equipment, biology, science projects, and teaching aids.

Tu-K Industries
5702 Firestone Place
South Gate, CA 90280
(800) 942-4TUK

All volumes of peroxide, containers, and disinfectants

American Association of Cosmetology Schools (AACS)
15825 N 71st Street, Suite 100
Scottsdale, AZ 85254
(800) 831-1086
www.beautyschool.org

One Roof
15825 N 71st Street, Suite 100
Scottsdale, AZ 85254
(800) 468-2274
www.oneroof.org

behindthechair.com
40 S Prospect, Suite 200
Roselle, IL 60172
(800) 760-3010
www.behindthechair.com

The Beauty and Barber Supply Institute, Inc. (BBSI)
15825 N 71st Street, Suite 100
Scottsdale, AZ 85254
(800) 468-BBSI
www.bbsi.org

The Salon Association (TSA)
15825 N 71st Street
Scottsdale, AZ 85254
(800) 211-4TSA
www.salons.org

International Cosmetology Expo (ICE)
15825 N 71st Street, Suite 100
Scottsdale, AZ 85254
(877) 442-3746 or (480) 281-0424 ext. 111
www.ice-shows.org

The Professional Beauty Federation (PBF)
15825 N 71st Street
Scottsdale, AZ 85254
(703) 527-7600, ext. 33
www.probeautyfederation.org

The National Cosmetology Association (NCA)
401 North Michigan Avenue
Chicago, IL 60611
(312) 527-6765
www.beautycity.com

Allured Publishing
362 South Schmale Road
Carol Stream, IL 60188
(630) 653-2155
CosmToil@allured.com
www.TheCosmeticSite.com

The Chemistry and Manufacture of Cosmetics, Volumes 1–3
Allured Publishing

Beginning Cosmetic Chemistry, Randy Schueller & Perry Ramanowski
Allured Publishing

Cosmetics and Toiletries Magazine
Allured Publishing

Global Cosmetic Industry Magazine
Advanstar Communications, Inc., Publisher
131 W. First Street
Duluth, MN 55802-2065
(800) 598-6008
www.advanstar.com

Global Cosmetic Industry Magazine
One Park Avenue
New York, NY 10016
www.globalcosmetic.com
www.cosmeticindex.com

The Society of Cosmetic Chemists (SCC)
120 Wall Street, Suite 2400
New York, NY 10005-4088
(212) 668-1500
www.scconline.org

The Society of Cosmetic Chemists, Monograph on *Permanent Hair Dyes*, Keith C. Brown and Stanley Pohl
The Society of Cosmetic Chemists, Monograph Number 7, *Skin, Hair and Nail Structure and Function and Associated Diseases*, Linda D. Rhein, Carolyn Peoples and Barbara Wolf

The Occupational Safety and Health Administration (OSHA)
(202) 693-1888
www.osha.gov

The U.S. Food and Drug Administration (FDA)
(202) 401-2242 or (202) 205-4706
http//vm.cfsan.fda.gov

Appendix E

Material Safety Data Sheets (MSDS)

Material Safety Data Sheets

MSDS:00013
Date Created:04/16/00
Worldwide Beauty Care
(Clairol, Inc.; Matrix Essentials, Inc.; Duart Labs; Redmond Products, Inc.)
Bristol-Myers Squibb Company
One Blachley Road
Stamford, CT 06922

Emergency Telephone Number:
(203) 357-5678

Transportation Emergency:
Call Chemtrec 1-800-424-9300

This sheet has been prepared in accordance with the Requirements of the OSHA Hazard Communication Standard, 29 CFR 1910.1200.

Section I - Categorization

Product Name: Permanent Wave Waving Lotions

Pertinent Text: Non-flammable water-like liquids containing ammonium thioglycolate with conditioners, preservatives and fragrance.

Product Names: Gentle Motion Waving Lotion, Opticolor Wave Waving Formula, Opticurl Waving Lotion, Perfecto Normal and Tinted Hair Waving Lotions, Synerfusion Waving Lotion, Systeme Biolage Acid Wave Waving Lotion, Therma-Vantage Controlled Exothermic Waving Lotions for Tinted and Normal Hair, VaVoom Volumizing Soft Wave Phase I

Section II - Ingredients Identity/Exposure Limits

Permanent Wave Waving Lotions generally contain the following hazardous ingredients (I% concentration or greater; 0.1% for carcinogens):

CTFA NAME	CAS#
AMMONIUM HYDROXIDE	1336216
EXPOSURE LIMIT: 25 PPM TLV, 35 PPM STEL, 50 PPM PEL, AS AMMONIA GLYCERIN	56815
EXPOSURE LIMIT: AS A MIST 10 MG/M'TLV, 15 MG/M'TOTAL; 5 MG/M'RESPIRABLE OSHA PEL	
ETHANOLAMINE	141435
EXPOSURE LIMIT: 3 PPM TLV, PEL, 6 PPM STEL AMMONIUM THIOGLYCOLATE	5421465
CYSTEINE HCL	52891
DIAMMONIUM DITHIODIGLYCOLATE	68223938
UREA57136	

Section III - Physical/Chemical Characteristics

Specific Gravity (H O = 1): 1.01-1.02　　　　pH: 8.5-9.0

Solubility in Water:　　Highly soluble.

Appearance and Odor: Yellowish water-like liquids. Slight ammoniacal and characteristic mercaptan thio odor.

Section IV - Fire and Explosion
Hazard Data

Flashpoint:　N/A　　　Unit:　N/A　　　Type:　Not applicable.
　　　　　　　　　　　Method: Not applicable.

Fire Fighting Procedures:
Extinguish fires with water ABC all-purpose or CO_2 extinguisher. The type of extinguisher used should be in conformance with local fire regulations.

Unusual Fire and Explosion Hazards:
On thermal decomposition can release hydrogen sulfide sulfur oxides and ammonia.

Figure E–1 *An example of a Material Safety Data Sheet* (MSDS) *for World Wide Beauty Care permanent waving solution (page I).*

Physical Hazards
None.
Section V–Reactivity Data

Stability:	Stable.
Conditions to Avoid:	Metallic bowls or stirrers.
Incompatibility (Materials to Avoid):	Heavy metals; oxidizing materials and acids.
Hazardous Decomposition or ByProducts:	Can release hydrogen sulfide; sulfur oxides and ammonia.

Section VI–Health Hazards and Hazard Data
The TLV of the mixture has not been established.
1. Effects of Acute Accidental Exposure
 Potential eye irritant.

Skin Contact:	Potential skin irritant.
Skin Sensitizer:	May induce hypersensitivity and elicit reactions in sensitized people.
Inhalation:	Respiratory tract irritant due to ammonia and mercaptan (thio) vapors.
Ingestion:	Moderately toxic.

2. Effects of Chronic Exposure   For purposes of chronic exposure under the OSHA Hazard Communication Standard this is an untested mixture. These products have been used extensively by consumers. Worldwide Beauty Care is not aware of any significant adverse reaction provided good work practices are observed (wash off skin, remove contaminated clothing, use good ventilation). Release of ammonia vapors may result in irritation of the mucous membranes of the respiratory tract. Published data indicate low level skin sensitization as a result of repeated heavy exposure principally in beauticians.

3. Carcinogen Status: OSHA: No   NTP: No   IARC: No

4. Route of Entry: Inhalation: Yes   Ingestion: Yes   Skin: Yes

5. Pre-existing dermatitis would likely be made worse by exposure to these products.

6. Emergency and First Aid Procedures

Eye Contact:	Remove contact lenses if used. Flush immediately with plenty of water for 15 minutes. Get medical attention IMMEDIATELY.
Skin Contact:	If spilled wash skin immediately with soap and water (do not use solvents). Change into clean clothing. If allergic reaction develops contact dermatologist.
Inhalation:	Remove person to fresh air. Increase ventilation.
Ingestion:	Rinse out mouth with water and administer large amounts of milk. Contact Employee Health Services immediately.

Section VII–Precautions for Safe Handling and Use
Steps to be taken in Case Material is released or Spilled:
Contain spill and promptly clean up. Flush with water and wipe with towel or rinse to drain. Floor can be slippery when wet.
Waste Disposal Method:
Disposal should be in accordance with all applicable local state and federal regulations.
Precautions to be Taken in Handling and Storage:
Store products in even normal temperatures. Keep containers tightly closed. Keep out of reach of children.

Section VIII–Control Measures

Ventilation:	Should be adequate to avoid concentration of irritating vapors.
Hand Protection:	Use impervious gloves to avoid possible skin irritation or sensitization.
Eye Protection:	Avoid contact with eyes. Use protective eyewear if splashing is possible.
Other Types of Protection:	None.
Respiratory Protection:	Avoid inhalation.
Work Hygienic Practices:	Always follow good hygienic work practices. Avoid all skin, eye, and clothing contact with products. In case of contact rinse thoroughly with water. Promptly clean up all spills.

Section IX–Transportation
Information
 DOT Class: Not regulated.   IMDG: Not regulated.   IATA/ICAO: Not regulated.

Figure E–2 *An example of a Material Safety Data Sheet (MSDS) for World Wide Beauty care permanent waving solution (page 2).*

Material Safety Data Sheet

MSDS: 00020
Date Approved: 11/1/2000

Worldwide Beauty Care
(Clairol, Inc.; Duart Labs; Redmond Products, Inc.)
Bristol-Myers Squibb Company
One Blachley Road
Stamford, CT 06922

Emergency Telephone Number:
(203) 357-5678

Transportation Emergency:
Call Chemtrec 1-800-424-9300

This sheet has been prepared in accordance with the Requirements of the OSHA Hazard Communication Standard, 29 CFR 1910.1200.

Section I - Categorization

Category: Relaxers.
Alkali metal hydroxides.
Product Names: Textures and Tones

Section II - Ingredients/Identity Exposure Limits
Relaxers generally contain the following hazardous ingredients (1% concentration or greater; 0.1% for carcinogens):

CTFA NAME	CAS#
PROPYLENE GLYCOL	57556
PETROLATUM	8027325
CETYL ALCOHOL	36653824
MINERAL OIL	8012951
EXPOSURE LIMIT: 5 mg/m^3 TLV, PEL as an Oil Mist	
POLYSORBATE 60	9005678
SODIUM HYDROXIDE	1310732
EXPOSURE LIMIT: C 2 mg/m^3, PEL	
CETEARYL ALCOHOL	67762270
CALCIUM HYDROXIDE	1305620
FRAGRANCE	999999999
POLYQUATERNIUM-28	98000022
GUANIDINE CARBONATE	593851

Section III - Physical/Chemical Characteristics
Specific Gravity (H$_2$O=1): Approximately 0.9
Solubility in Water: Partly miscible.
Appearance and Odor: Thick, white cremes with fragranced odor.

pH: N/A

TRADE
MSDS #20

Page 1 of 3

Figure E-3 *An example of a Material Safety Data Sheet (MSDS) for alkali metal hydroxide hair relaxers (page 1).*

Section IV - Fire and Explosion Hazard Data

Flashpoint: N/A   **Unit:** N/A

Type: Not applicable.   **Method:** Not applicable.

Fire Fighting Procedures:
Extinguish fires with ABC all-purpose extinguisher. The type of extinguisher used should be in conformance with local fire regulations. Fire fighters should use self contained breathing apparatus in enclosed areas.

Unusual Fire and Explosion Hazards:
None.

Physical Hazards:
None.

Section V - Reactivity Data

Stability:	Stable.
Conditions to Avoid:	Heat and sunlight.
Incompatibility (Materials to Avoid):	Acids; metal containers.
Hazardous Decomposition or By Products:	None.

Section VI - Health Hazards and Hazard Data

The TLV of the mixture has not been established.

1. Effects of Acute Accidental Exposure

Eye Contact:
Severe eye irritant. CORROSIVE.

Skin Contact:
CORROSIVE.

Inhalation:
Not likely to be inhaled.

Ingestion:
Will result in severe irritation to mouth, esophagus and gastrointestinal tract.

2. Effects of Chronic Exposure

For purposes of chronic exposure under the OSHA Hazard Communication Standard, this is an untested mixture. No chronic adverse effects are expected. Target Organs: These products contain an ingredient which have been shown to affect tissues or organs under high levels of exposure in animal studies not encountered in normal use. Propylene Glycol: Kidney.

3. Carcinogen Status:

   OSHA: No   NTP: No   IARC: No

4. Route of Entry:

   Inhalation: No   Ingestion: Yes   Skin: Yes

5. Pre-existing dermatitis would likely be made worse by exposure to these products.

Figure E-4 *An example of a* Material Safety Data Sheet (MSDS) *for alkali metal hydroxide hair relaxers (page 2).*

6. Emergency and First Aid Procedures

Eye Contact:
Remove contact lenses, if used. Flush immediately with plenty of water for 15 minutes. Get medical attention IMMEDIATELY.

Skin Contact:
If spilled, wash skin immediately with soap and water (do not use solvents). Change into clean clothing. If skin reaction develops, contact dermatologist.

Inhalation:
Remove person to fresh air. Increase ventilation.

Ingestion:
Rinse out mouth with water and administer large amounts of milk. Contact Poison Control Center.

Section VII - Precautions for Safe Handling and Use

Steps to be taken in Case Material is released or Spilled:
Contain spill and promptly clean up. Flush with water and wipe with towel or rinse to drain. Floor can be slippery when wet.

Waste Disposal Method:
Products covered by this MSDS, in their original form, are considered non-hazardous waste according to RCRA. Additionally, disposal should be in accordance with all applicable Local, State and Federal Regulations.

Precautions to be Taken in Handling and Storage:
Store products in even, normal temperatures. Keep containers tightly closed.

Section VIII - Control Measures

Ventilation:
Exhaust system ventilation should be adequate to avoid buildup of vapors.

Hand Protection:
CORROSIVE. Use impervious gloves to avoid possible skin irritation or sensitization.

Eye Protection:
Severely irritating/corrosive. Avoid contact with eyes.

Other Types of Protection:
Not applicable.

Respiratory Protection:
Avoid inhalation.

Work Hygienic Practices:
Always follow good hygienic work practices. Avoid eye, clothing, and prolonged skin contact with products. In case of contact, rinse thoroughly with water. Promptly clean up all spills.

Section IX - Transportation Information

DOT Class: Consumer Commodity ORMD up to 2-1/1 lbs., Over 2-1/2 lbs: Corrosive solid, basic, organic, N.O.S., 8, UN3263, PGII, (Contains Sodium Hydroxide).

IMDG: Corrosive Solid Basic Organic N.O.S., (Contains Sodium Hydroxide), 8, UN 3263, PGII

IATA/ICAO: Corrosive Solid, Basic, Organic, n.o.s. (contains sodium hydroxide) 8, UN3263, Packing Instruction: Passenger Aircraft 814 II Cargo Aircraft 816 II

TRADE
MSDS #20   **Page 3 of 3**

Figure E–5 *An example of a Material Safety Data Sheet* (MSDS) *for alkali metal hydroxide hair relaxers (page 3).*

Kenra, LLC 6501 Julian Ave., Indianapolis, IN 46219

Product Name	QP BLACK INDIGO COLOR
Product Description	Color
MSDS Number: 560804	**Revision Date:** 17-Jul-00

ELASTA
PRODUCTS COMPANY

Section 2 - Hazardous Ingredients / Identity Information

Hazardous Components	CAS Number	TLV or PEL	Other Limits	Percentage
None	N/A	N/A	N/A	N/A

Section 3 - Physical/Chemical Characteristics

Boiling Point	N/A	**Specific Gravity H20 = 1**	1.005
Vapor Pressure (mm Hg.)	N/A	**Melting Point**	N/A
Vapor Density (AIR = 1)	N/A	**Evaporation Point(Butyl Acetate = 1)**	N/A
Solubility in Water	Semi		
Appearance and Odor	Bluish black opaque / neutral odor.		

Section 4 - Fire and Expolsion Hazard

Flash Point (Method Used)	Flammable Limits	LEL	UEL
N/A	N/A	N/A	N/A

Extinguishing Media

All purpose extinguisher.

Special Fire Fighting Procedures

N/A

Unusual Fire and Explosion Hazards

N/A

Section 5 - Reactvity Data

Stability	Unstable ☐	**Conditions to Avoid**
	Stable ☑	N/A

Incompatibilty (Materials to Avoid)

N/A

Hazardous Decomposition or Byproducts

N/A

Hazardous Polymerization	May Occur ☐	**Conditions to Avoid**
	May Not Occur ☑	N/A

Figure E-6 *An example of a Material Safety Data Sheet (MSDS) for semi-permanent haircolor.*
(Reprinted with permission of Kenra LLC.)

Material Safety Data Sheet-PPD

MSDS:0001C
Date Approved:
Worldwide Beauty Care
(Clairol, Inc.; Duart Labs; Redmond Products, Inc.)
Bristol-Myers Squibb Company
One Blachley Road
Stamford, CT 06922

Emergency Telephone Number:	**Transportation Emergency:**
(203) 357-5678	Call Chemtrec 1-800-424-9300

This sheet has been prepared in accordance with the Requirements of the OSHA Hazard Communication Standard, 29 CFR 1910.1200.

▼

Section I - Categorization
Product Category: Ammoniacal Oxidation (Permanent) Hair Colors, Flammable
Pertinent Text: Oxidation Hair Colors contain low concentrations of dye intermediates in an aqueous base. They are mixed with the developer (hydrogen peroxide) before use. A separate MSDS exists for hydrogen peroxide.
Product Names: Miss Clairol, Summer Blonde Lightener, Complements Gel Color Permanent, Creme Toner

▼

Section II - Ingredients Identity/Exposure Limits
Ammoniacal Oxidation (Permanent) Hair Colors, Flammable generally contain the following hazardous ingredients (1% concentration or greater; 0.1% for carcinogens):

CTFA Name	CAS Number
M-AMINOPHENOL	591275
N,N-BIS(2-HYDROXYETHYL)-P-PHENYLENEDIAMINE SULFATE	58262445
RESORCINOL	108463
EXPOSURE LIMIT:10 ppm TLV, 20 ppm STEL	
P-PHENYLENEDIAMINE	106503
EXPOSURE LIMIT:0.1 mg/m3 TLV, PEL, SKIN, OSHA	
PROPYLENE GLYCOL	57556
AMMONIUM HYDROXIDE	1336216
EXPOSURE LIMIT:25 ppm TLV, 35 ppm STEL, 50 ppm PEL, as AMMONIA	
ETHOXYDIGLYCOL	111900
ETHANOLAMINE	141435
EXPOSURE LIMIT:3 ppm TLV, PEL, 6 ppm STEL	
NONOXYNOL-4	7311275
OLEALKONIUM CHLORIDE	37139994
HEXYLENE GLYCOL	107415
EXPOSURE LIMIT:25 ppm CEILING ACGIH	
OLEIC ACID	112801
STEARYL ALCOHOL	112925
SOYTRIMONIUM CHLORIDE	61790418
ISOPROPYL ALCOHOL	67630
EXPOSURE LIMIT:400 ppm TLV, PEL, 500 ppm STEL	
NONOXYNOL-2	27176938
LAURYL ALCOHOL	112538
4-AMINO-2-HYDROXYTOLUENE	2835952
STEARETH-21	977080811
PEG-15 COCOPOLYAMINE	977159208
COCAMIDE MEA	68140001

Figure E-7 *An example of a Material Safety Data Sheet (MSDS) for permanent oxidation haircolors with ammonia (page 1).*

(Reprinted with permission of Clairol Inc.)

PEG-3 DIOLEOYLAMIDOETHYLMONIUM METHOSULFATE	98000176
FRAGRANCE	999999999
STEARETH-21	977080811
PROPYLENE GLYCOL	57556
SOYTRIMONIUM CHLORIDE	61790418
OLEAMIDE MIPA	111057
POLYQUATERNIUM-22	53694170
CYCLOMETHICONE	69430246
DIHYDROXYETHYL TALLOW GLYCINATE	61791455
GLYCERIN	56815

EXPOSURE LIMIT:AS A MIST 10 mg/m3 TLV, 15 mg/m3 TOTAL: 5 mg/m3 RESPIRABLE OSHA PEL

OCTOXYNOL-1   2315675

Section III - Physical/Chemical Characteristics

Specific Gravity (H$_2$O = 1):	0.995 -1.009	pH:	9.5 - 10.8
Solubility in Water:	Partly soluble.	Appearance and Odor:	Fragranced liquids. Ammoniacal odor.

Section IV - Fire and Explosion Hazard Data

Flashpoint:	<100^0	Unit:	Fahrenheit	Type:	For products containing alcohol.
		Method:	closed cup		

Fire Fighting Procedures:
Extinguish fires with ABC all-purpose extinguisher. The type of extinguisher used should be in conformance with local fire regulations. Fire fighters should use self contained breathing apparatus in enclosed areas.

Unusual Fire and Explosion Hazards:
Not applicable.

Physical Hazards
According to OSHA,these products are considered to be flammable.

Section V - Reactivity Data

Stability:	Stable.
Conditions to Avoid:	Heat and sunlight.
Incompatibility (Materials ot Avoid):	Acids.
Hazardous Decomposition or ByProducts:	May form toxic materials (carbon dioxide,carbon monoxide and ammonia).

Section VI- Health Hazards and Hazard Data

The TLV of the mixture has not been established.

1. Effects of Acute Accidental Exposure

Eye Contact:	CAUTION. Unmixed oxidation haircolors are eye irritants. When oxidation haircolors are mixed with developers (hydrogen peroxide),the mixture may cause severe irritation and possible permanent eye injury.
Skin Contact:	May cause skin irritation or sensitization in sensitized individuals.
Inhalation:	Inhalation of ammonia vapors may result in respiratory irritation.
Ingestion:	Moderately toxic.

2. Effects of Chronic Exposure
A composite mixture of oxidation dyes has been tested in prolonged topical exposure studies of laboratory animals. No adverse effects on growth, reproduction or general health were observed. In topical studies no target

Figure E-8 *An example of a Material Safety Data Sheet (MSDS) for permanent oxidation haircolors with ammonia (page 2).*

(Reprinted with permission of Clairol Inc.)

organ toxicity was observed other than limited effect on treated skin.

3. Carcinogen Status:
OSHA: No NTP: No IARC: No

4. Route of Entry:
Inhalation: Yes Ingestion: Yes Skin: Yes

5. Pre-existing dermatitis would likely be made worse by exposure to these products.

6. Emergency and First Aid Procedures

Eye Contact: Remove contact lenses. Flush immediately with plenty of water for 15 minutes. Get medical attention IMMEDIATELY.

Skin Contact: If spilled,wash skin immediately with soap and water (do not use solvents). Change into clean clothing. If skin irritation or sensitization develops,contact dermatologist.

Inhalation: Remove person to fresh air. Increase ventilation.

Ingestion: Rinse out mouth with water and administer large amounts of milk. Contact Poison Control Center.

Section VII - Precautions for Safe Handling and Use

Steps to be taken in Case Material is released or Spilled:
Contain spill and promptly clean up. Flush with water and wipe with towel or rinse to drain. Floor can be slippery when wet.

Waste Disposal Method:
Products covered by this MSDS,in their original form,are considered non-hazardous waste according to RCRA (40 CFR 261.21(1)). Additionally,disposal should be in accordance with all applicable Local,State and Federal regulations.

Precautions to be Taken in Handling and Storage:
Follow flammable liquid handling and storage requirements. Do not store any haircolor after it has been mixed with developer. Decomposition of hydrogen peroxide may occur with increase in pressure and possible container rupture. Keep away from heat and other ignition sources.

Section VIII - Control Measures

Ventilation:
Exhaust system ventilation should be adequate to avoid buildup of vapors.

Hand Protection:
Use impervious gloves to avoid possible skin irritation/sensitization.

Eye Protection:
Avoid contact with eyes. Use protective eyewear,if splashing is possible.

Other Types of Protection:
Not applicable.

Respiratory Protection:
Avoid inhalation.

Work Hygienic Practices:
Always follow good hygienic work practices. Avoid all skin,eye,and clothing contact with products. In case of contact,rinse thoroughly with water. Promptly clean up all spills.

Section IX - Transportation Information

DOT Class: Consumer Commodity ORM-D	**IMDG:**Ethanol Solutions (Limited Quantity) 3.3 UN1170, PGIII (Flash Point)	**IATA/ICAO:**Consumer Commodity Class: 9, ID 8000 Packing Instruction 910

Figure E-9 *An example of a Material Safety Data Sheet (MSDS) for permanent oxidation haircolors with ammonia (page 3).*

(Reprinted with permission of Clairol Inc.)

Material Safety Data Sheet-PPD

MSDS:0001F-1
Date Approved:
Worldwide Beauty Care
(Clairol, Inc.; Duart Labs; Redmond Products, Inc.)
Bristol-Myers Squibb Company
One Blachley Road
Stamford, CT 06922

Emergency Telephone Number:	**Transportation Emergency:**
(203) 357-5678	Call Chemtrec 1-800-424-9300

This sheet has been prepared in accordance with the Requirements of the OSHA Hazard Communication Standard, 29 CFR 1910.1200.

▼

Section I - Categorization
Product Category: Oxidation (Permanent) Hair Colors - Non-Ammonia-Non -Flammable
Pertinent Text:
Product Names: Radiance Color Gloss

▼

Section II - Ingredients Identity/Exposure Limits
Oxidation (Permanent) Hair Colors - Non-Ammonia-Non -Flammable generally contain the following hazardous ingredients (1% concentration or greater; 0.1% for carcinogens):

CTFA Name	CAS Number
M-AMINOPHENOL	591275
N,N-BIS(2-HYDROXYETHYL)-P-PHENYLENEDIAMINE SULFATE	58262445
2-NITRO-P-PHENYLENEDIAMINE	5307142
RESORCINOL	108463
EXPOSURE LIMIT:10 ppm TLV, 20 ppm STEL	
P-PHENYLENEDIAMINE	106503
EXPOSURE LIMIT:0.1 mg/m3 TLV, PEL, SKIN, OSHA	
ETHOXYDIGLYCOL	111900
LAURETH-23	9002920
POLYSORBATE 20	9005645
NONYL NONOXYNOL-49	9014931A
OLEIC ACID	112801
AMINOMETHYL PROPANOL	124685
2-METHYLRESORCINOL	608253
DIHYDROXYPROPYL PEG-5 LINOLEAMMONIUM CHLORIDE	98000070
AMODIMETHICONE	977091647

▼

Section III - Physical/Chemical Characteristics

Specific Gravity (H$_2$O = 1):0.995-1.009		**pH:**	9.5-10.5
Solubility in Water:	Partly soluble.	**Appearance and Odor:**	Fragranced liquids.

▼

Section IV - Fire and Explosion
Hazard Data

Flashpoint:	Not applicable.	**Unit:**	N/A	**Type:**Not applicable.	
		Method:	Not applicable.		

Fire Fighting Procedures:
Extinguish fires with water,ABC all-purpose or C02 extinguisher. The type of extinguisher used should be in conformance with local fire regulations.

Figure E-10 *An example of a Material Safety Data Sheet (MSDS) for permanent oxidation haircolors without ammonia (page 1).*

(Reprinted with permission of Clairol Inc.)

Unusual Fire and Explosion Hazards:
Not applicable.
Physical Hazards
None.

Section V - Reactivity Data

Stability:	Stable.
Conditions to Avoid:	Heat and sunlight.
Incompatibility (Materials ot Avoid):	Acids.
Hazardous Decomposition or ByProducts:	None.

Section VI- Health Hazards and Hazard Data

The TLV of the mixture has not been established.

1. Effects of Acute Accidental Exposure

Eye Contact:	CAUTION. Unmixed oxidation haircolors are eye irritants. When oxidation haircolors are mixed with developers (hydrogen peroxide),the mixture may cause severe irritation and possible permanent eye injury.
Skin Contact:	May cause skin irritation or sensitization in sensitized individuals.
Inhalation:	Inhalation of vapors may result in respiratory irritation.
Ingestion:	Moderately toxic.

2. Effects of Chronic Exposure

These products contain 2-nitro-p-phenylenediamine, which fed at extremely high doses, were found to cause benign liver tumors in female mice (NTP). These effects were not observed in feeding studies in male mice or male and female rats. Independent pathologists and oncologists have concluded that the results are not relevant to human health. In topical studies no target organ toxicity was observed other than limited effects on treated skin.

3. Carcinogen Status:

OSHA: No NTP: Yes (2 Nitro PPD) IARC: 2 Nitro PPD is not Classifiable (Group 3)

4. Route of Entry:

Inhalation: No Ingestion: Yes Skin: Yes

5. Pre-existing dermatitis would likely be made worse by exposure to these products. Bronchitis may be aggravated by irritant vapors.

6. Emergency and First Aid Procedures

Eye Contact:	Remove contact lenses,if used. Flush immediately with plenty of water for 15 minutes. Get medical attention IMMEDIATELY.
Skin Contact:	If spilled,wash skin immediately with soap and water (do not use solvents). Change into clean clothing. If skin irritation or sensitization develops,contact dermatologist.
Inhalation:	Remove person to fresh air. Increase ventilation.
Ingestion:	Rinse out mouth with water and administer large amounts of milk. Contact Poison Control Center.

Section VII - Precautions for Safe Handling and Use

Steps to be taken in Case Material is released or Spilled:
Contain spill and promptly clean up. Flush with water and wipe with towel or rinse to drain. Floor can be slippery when wet.

Waste Disposal Method:
Products covered by this MSDS,in their original form,are considered non-hazardous waste according to RCRA. Additionally,disposal should be in accordance with all applicable Local,State and Federal regulations.

Precautions to be Taken in Handling and Storage:
Do not expose to sunlight. Keep away from radiators and heat. Do not store any haircolor after it has been mixed with developer. Decomposition of hydrogen peroxide may occur with increase in pressure and possible container rupture.

Section VIII - Control Measures

Ventilation:
Exhaust system ventilation should be adequate to avoid buildup of vapors.

Hand Protection:
Use impervious gloves to avoid possible skin irritation/sensitization.

Eye Protection:

Figure E-11 *An example of a Material Safety Data Sheet (MSDS) for permanent oxidation haircolors without ammonia (page 2).*

(Reprinted with permission of Clairol Inc.)

Avoid contact with eyes. Use protective eyewear,if splashing is possible.
Other Types of Protection:
Not applicable.
Respiratory Protection:
Avoid inhalation.
Work Hygienic Practices:
Always follow good hygienic work practices. Avoid all skin,eye,and clothing contact with products. In case of contact,rinse thoroughly with water. Promptly clean up all spills.

Section IX - Transportation Information

DOT Class: Not regulated.	**IMDG:**Not regulated.	**IATA/ICAO:**Not regulated.

Figure E-12 *An example of a Material Safety Data Sheet (MSDS) for permanent oxidation haircolors without ammonia (page 3).*

(Reprinted with permission of Clairol Inc.)

Material Safety Data Sheet

MSDS: 00002-1
Date Approved: 11/1/2000

Worldwide Beauty Care
(Clairol, Inc.; Duart Labs; Redmond Products, Inc.)
Bristol-Myers Squibb Company
One Blachley Road
Stamford, CT 06922

Emergency Telephone Number:	**Transportation Emergency:**
(203) 357-5678	Call Chemtrec 1-800-424-9300

This sheet has been prepared in accordance with the Requirements of the OSHA Hazard Communication Standard, 29 CFR 1910.1200.

Section I - Categorization

Category: Semipermanent Hair Colors.
Non- ammoniacal hair dye formulations used without peroxide.
Product Names: Silk & Silver Shades

Section II - Ingredients/Identity Exposure Limits
Semipermanent Hair Colors generally contain the following hazardous ingredients (1% concentration or greater; 0.1% for carcinogens):

CTFA NAME	CAS#
ETHOXYDIGLYCOL	111900
HYDROXYETHYLCELLULOSE	9004620
OLEIC ACID	112801
PEG-50 TALLOW AMIDE	8051636
AMINOMETHYL PROPANOL	124685
HC BLUE NO. 2	33229344
TRIMETHYLSILYLAMODIMETHICONE	977088826
LAURAMIDE DEA	120401

Section III - Physical/Chemical Characteristics
Specific Gravity (H₂O=1): 0.992 -1.997   pH: 8.3-9.3
Solubility in Water: Miscible.
Appearance and Odor: Clear fragranced amber liquid.

Figure E-13 *An example of a Material Safety Data Sheet (MSDS) for semi-permanent non-oxidation haircolors, without peroxide or ammonia (page 1).*

(Reprinted with permission of Clairol Inc.)

Section IV - Fire and Explosion Hazard Data

Flashpoint: > 200⁰

Type: Not applicable.

Unit: Fahrenheit

Method: closed cup

Fire Fighting Procedures:

Extinguish fires with ABC all-purpose extinguisher. The type of extinguisher used should be in conformance with local fire regulations. Fire fighters should use self-contained breathing apparatus in enclosed areas.

Unusual Fire and Explosion Hazards:

None.

Physical Hazards:

None.

Section V - Reactivity Data

Stability:	Stable.
Conditions to Avoid:	Heat and sunlight.
Incompatibility (Materials to Avoid):	Not applicable.
Hazardous Decomposition or By Products:	None.

Section VI - Health Hazards and Hazard Data

The TLV of the mixture has not been established.

1. Effects of Acute Accidental Exposure

Eye Contact:

CAUTION. Eye irritant.

Skin Contact:

May cause skin irritation or sensitization in sensitized individuals.

Inhalation:

Not likely to be irritating.

Ingestion:

Moderately toxic.

2. Effects of Chronic Exposure

National Toxicology Program studies on diethanolamine (DEA), itself and fatty acid condensates containing free diethanolamine (lauramide and cocamide diethanolamines), indicated an increased incidence of kidney and/or liver tumors in mice dermally exposed for their lifetime. The significance of these findings and their potential relevance to humans are not clear and further studies are in progress. Diethanolamine or its condensates did not induce tumors in rats. In the interim, the U.S. CIR, which had previously considered these materials as "safe as used", has expressed reservation over NTP's conclusions and saw no need to revise its conclusions until several outstanding questions on the NTP methodology are answered.

The semipermanent dye products have been tested in lifetime skin painting studies on laboratory animals. No adverse effects on growth, reproduction or general health were observed. In topical studies, other than limited effect on treated skin, no target organ toxicity was observed to any organ.

3. Carcinogen Status:

OSHA: No   NTP: Yes (DEAs)   IARC: DEA is not Classifiable (Group 3)

4. Route of Entry:

Inhalation: No   Ingestion: Yes   Skin: Yes

5. Pre-existing dermatitis would likely be made worse by exposure to these products.

Figure E-14 *An example of a Material Safety Data Sheet (MSDS) for semi-permanent non-oxidation haircolors, without peroxide or ammonia (page 1).*

(Reprinted with permission of Clairol Inc.)

Section VI – Health Hazards and Hazard Data (Continued)

6. Emergency and First Aid Procedures
Eye Contact:
Remove contact lenses, if used. Flush immediately with plenty of water for 15 minutes. Get medical attention IMMEDIATELY.
Skin Contact:
If spilled, wash skin immediately with soap and water (do not use solvents). Change into clean clothing. If skin irritation or sensitization develops, contact dermatologist.
Inhalation:
Remove person to fresh air. Increase ventilation.
Ingestion:
Rinse out mouth with water and administer large amounts of milk. Contact Poison Control Center.

Section VII - Precautions for Safe Handling and Use
Steps to be taken in Case Material is released or Spilled:
Contain spill and promptly clean up. Flush with water and wipe with towel or rinse to drain. Floor can be slippery when wet.
Waste Disposal Method:
Products covered by this MSDS, in their original form, are considered non-hazardous waste according to RCRA. Additionally, disposal should be in accordance with Local, State and Federal Regulations.
Precautions to be Taken in Handling and Storage:
Do not expose to sunlight. Keep away from radiators and heat.

Section VIII - Control Measures
Ventilation:
Exhaust system ventilation should be adequate to avoid buildup of vapors.
Hand Protection:
Use impervious gloves to avoid possible skin irritation/sensitization.
Eye Protection:
Avoid contact with eyes. Use protective eyewear, if splashing is possible.
Other Types of Protection:
Not applicable.
Respiratory Protection:
Avoid inhalation.
Work Hygienic Practices:
Always follow good hygienic work practices. Avoid all skin, eye, and clothing contact with products. In case of contact, rinse thoroughly with water. Promptly clean up all spills.

Section IX - Transportation Information
DOT Class: Not regulated.
IMDG: Not regulated.
IATA/ICAO: Not regulated.

Figure E-15 *An example of a Material Safety Data Sheet (MSDS) for semi-permanent non-oxidation haircolors, without peroxide or ammonia (page 2).*

(Reprinted with permission of Clairol Inc.)

Material Safety Data Sheet-PPD

MSDS:00006
Date Approved:
Worldwide Beauty Care
(Clairol, Inc.; Duart Labs; Redmond Products, Inc.)
Bristol-Myers Squibb Company
One Blachley Road
Stamford, CT 06922

Emergency Telephone Number: **Transportation Emergency:**
(203) 357-5678   Call Chemtrec 1-800-424-9300

This sheet has been prepared in accordance with the Requirements of the OSHA Hazard Communication Standard, 29 CFR 1910.1200.

▼

Section I - Categorization
Product Category: Lightener Lotions

Pertinent Text: Hair lighteners are composed of lightener lotions that are mixed with hydrogen peroxide (developers). A third component is often added to accelerate the lightening. These are called either protinators or accelerators and they are found under the category of Bleach Powders. This MSDS covers Lightener Lotions. Consult separate MSDS's for bleach powder and hydrogen peroxide (developers).

Product Names: Born Blonde Liquid Lightener, 7th Stage Liquid Lightener, Complements Lightening Gel, Instant Whip Liquid Lightener, Maxi Blonde Lightener, Ultra Blue Creme Lightener, Ultra Blue Lady Clairol Lightener, Xtreme FX Bleach-Out Lotion Lightener, Frost & Tip Highlightening Powder, BW Violet Creme Lightener

▼

Section II - Ingredients Identity/Exposure Limits
Lightener Lotions generally contain the following hazardous ingredients (1% concentration or greater; 0.1% for carcinogens):

CTFA Name	CAS Number
PROPYLENE GLYCOL	57556
AMMONIUM HYDROXIDE	1336216
EXPOSURE LIMIT:25 ppm TLV, 35 ppm STEL, 50 ppm PEL, as AMMONIA	
ISOPROPYL ALCOHOL	67630
EXPOSURE LIMIT:400 ppm TLV, PEL, 500 ppm STEL	
ETHOXYDIGLYCOL	111900
GLYCERIN	56815
EXPOSURE LIMIT:AS A MIST 10 mg/m3 TLV, 15 mg/m3 TOTAL; 5 mg/m3 RESPIRABLE OSHA PEL	
PHOSPHORIC ACID	7664382
EXPOSURE LIMIT:1 mg/m3 TLV, PEL, 3 mg/m3 STEL	
TRIDECETH-6	24938918
NONYL NONOXYNOL-10	9014931G
ETHANOLAMINE	141435
EXPOSURE LIMIT:3 ppm TLV, PEL, 6 ppm STEL	
OCTOXYNOL-1	2315675
NONOXYNOL-4	7311275
PEG-5 SOYAMINE	61791240G
SULFATED CASTOR OIL	8002333
PEG-8 HYDROGENATED TALLOW AMINE	61791262G
HEXYLENE GLYCOL	107415
EXPOSURE LIMIT:25 ppm CEILING ACGIH	
OLETH-20	9004982
NONYL NONOXYNOL-49	9014931A
CETYL ALCOHOL	36653824
ALCOHOL DENAT.	64175

Figure E-16 *An example of a Material Safety Data Sheet (MSDS) hair lightener lotions (page 1).*
(Reprinted with permission of Clairol Inc.)

EXPOSURE LIMIT:1000 ppm TLV, PEL (ETHYL ALCOHOL)

OLEIC ACID	112801
SODIUM LAURYL SULFATE	151213
ETHYL HYDROXYMETHYL OLEYL OXAZOLINE	68140987
PPG-50 CETYL ETHER	9035852
COCETH-7 CARBOXYLIC ACID	977159424
STEARETH-21	977080811
OLETH-20	9004982
PEG-15 COCOPOLYAMINE	977159208
DIMETHICONE COPOLYOL	64365237
SODIUM LAURETH-13 CARBOXYLATE	33939649G
SODIUM LAURETH-11 CARBOXYLATE	33939649
DILINOLEIC ACID	6144281
C12-15 PARETH-3	98000085

▼

Section III - Physical/Chemical Characteristics

Specific Gravity (H$_2$O = 1): 0.9-1.1   **pH:** N/A

Solubility in Water: Fairly miscible (thickens with water).   **Appearance and Odor:** Fragranced, pourable emulsions. Ammoniacal odor.

Section IV - Fire and Explosion Hazard Data

Flashpoint: 75 - 104   **Unit:** Fahrenheit   **Type:** For products containing alcohol.

Method: closed cup

Fire Fighting Procedures:
Extinguish fires with water, ABC all-purpose or C02 extinguisher. The type of extinguisher used should be in conformance with local fire regulations. Fire fighters should use self contained breathing apparatus in enclosed areas.

Unusual Fire and Explosion Hazards:
None.

Physical Hazards
Products containing alcohol are usually flammable or combustible liquids.

Section V - Reactivity Data

Stability: Stable.
Conditions to Avoid: Heat and sunlight.
Incompatibility (Materials ot Avoid): Do not use metallic bowls or stirrers.
Hazardous Decomposition or ByProducts: None.

Section VI- Health Hazards and Hazard Data
The TLV of the mixture has not been established.
1. Effects of Acute Accidental Exposure

Eye Contact: CAUTION. Eye irritants. When the lightener lotion is mixed with hydrogen peroxide, the mixture may cause severe irritation and possible permanent eye injury.
Skin Contact: Irritant. May induce a skin reaction in certain individuals.
Inhalation: Ammonia vapor may cause respiratory tract irritation.
Ingestion: Moderately toxic.

Figure E-17 *An example of a Material Safety Data Sheet (MSDS) hair lightener lotions (page 2).*
(Reprinted with permission of Clairol Inc.)

2. Effects of Chronic Exposure

For purposes of chronic exposure under the OSHA Hazard Communication Standard, this is an untested mixture. These products have been used extensively by consumers and Worldwide Beauty Care is not aware of any significant adverse effects. Release of ammonia vapors may result in irritation of the mucous membranes of the respiratory tract. Target Organs: These products contain ingredients which have been shown to affect tissues or organs when fed at high levels to animals. Exposure from professional uses of these products is well below the exposure levels used in animal studies. Target organs identified in animal studies are as follows: Glycerin: Kidney Liver; Isopropyl Alcohol: CNS; SD Alcohol 40: Liver, Eye, CNS, Reproductive; Propylene Glycol: CNS

3. Carcinogen Status:

OSHA: No NTP: No IARC: No

4. Route of Entry:

Inhalation: No Ingestion: Yes Skin: Yes

5. Pre-existing dermatitis would likely be made worse by exposure to these products.

6. Emergency and First Aid Procedures

Eye Contact:	Remove contact lenses, if used. Flush immediately with plenty of water for 15 minutes. Get medical attention IMMEDIATELY.
Skin Contact:	If spilled, wash skin immediately with soap and water (do not use solvents). Change into clean clothing. If skin reaction develops, contact dermatologist.
Inhalation:	Remove person to fresh air. Increase ventilation.
Ingestion:	Rinse out mouth with water and administer large amounts of milk. Contact Poison Control Center.

Section VII - Precautions for Safe Handling and Use

Steps to be taken in Case Material is released or Spilled:

Contain spill and promptly clean up. Flush with water and wipe with towel or rinse to drain. Floor can be slippery when wet.

Waste Disposal Method:

Products covered by this MSDS, in their original form, are considered non-hazardous waste according to RCRA (4 CFR 261.21(1)). Additionally, disposal should be in accordance with all applicable Local, State and Federal regulations.

Precautions to be Taken in Handling and Storage:

Do not store any lightener lotion after it has been mixed with developer and bleach powder. Decomposition of hydrogen peroxide may occur with increase in pressure and possible container rupture.

Section VIII - Control Measures

Ventilation:

Exhaust system ventilation should be adequate to avoid buildup of vapors.

Hand Protection:

Use impervious gloves to avoid possible skin irritation or sensitization.

Eye Protection:

Avoid contact with eyes. Use protective eyewear, if splashing is possible.

Other Types of Protection:

Not applicable.

Respiratory Protection:

Avoid inhalation.

Work Hygienic Practices:

Always follow good hygienic work practices. Avoid all skin, eye, and clothing contact with products. In case of contact, rinse thoroughly with water. Promptly clean up all spills.

Section IX - Transportation Information

DOT Class: Consumer Commodity ORM-D	**IMDG:** Ethanol Solutions 3.3 UN1170, PGIII (75-104F) Limited Quantity	**IATA/ICAO:** Consumer Commodity Class: 9, ID 800 Packing Instructions 910

Figure E-18 *An example of a Material Safety Data Sheet (MSDS) hair lightener lotions (page 3).*

(Reprinted with permission of Clairol Inc.)

Material Safety Data Sheet-PPD

MSDS:00007-1
Date Approved:
Worldwide Beauty Care
(Clairol, Inc.; Duart Labs; Redmond Products, Inc.)
Bristol-Myers Squibb Company
One Blachley Road
Stamford, CT 06922

Emergency Telephone Number:	**Transportation Emergency:**
(203) 357-5678	Call Chemtrec 1-800-424-9300

This sheet has been prepared in accordance with the Requirements of the OSHA Hazard Communication Standard, 29 CFR 1910.1200.

▼
Section I - Categorization
Product Category: Shampoos
Pertinent Text: Viscous colored liquids or emulsions containing surfactants to cleanse the hair.
Product Names: Texture & TonesMoisturizing Shampoo, Complements Maintenance Shampoo, Condition 3-In-1 Shampoos, Daily Defense Shampoos, Shimmer Lights Shampoo

▼
Section II - Ingredients Identity/Exposure Limits
Shampoos generally contain the following hazardous ingredients (1% concentration or greater; 0.1% for carcinogens):

CTFA Name	CAS Number
GLYCERIN	56815
EXPOSURE LIMIT:AS A MIST 10 mg/m3 TLV, 15 mg/m3 TOTAL: 5 mg/m3 RESPIRABLE OSHA PEL	
SALICYLIC ACID	69727
SODIUM CHLORIDE	7647145
COCAMIDE DEA	61791319
LAURAMIDE DEA	120401
SODIUM CITRATE	68042
ALCOHOL DENAT.	64175
EXPOSURE LIMIT:1000 PPM TLV, PEL (ETHYL ALCOHOL)	
DISODIUM COCOAMPHODIACETATE	68650395
SODIUM LAURYL SULFATE	151213
AMMONIUM LAURYL SULFATE	2235543
DISODIUM COCAMIDO MIPA-SULFOSUCCINATE	68515651
DISODIUM COCOAMPHODIACETATE	68650395
GLYCOL STEARATE	111604
SODIUM LAUROYL SARCOSINATE	137166
COCAMIDOPROPYL BETAINE	61789400
SODIUM C14-16 OLEFIN SULFONATE	68439576
LAURAMIDE DEA	120401
SODIUM LAURETH SULFATE	1335724
PEG-120 METHYL GLUCOSE DIOLEATE	86893198
TEA-LAURYL SULFATE	139968
PEG-15 COCOPOLYAMINE	977159208
COCAMIDE MEA	68140001
SODIUM LAURYL SULFATE	151213
FRAGRANCE	999999999
PROPYLENE GLYCOL	57556
LINOLEAMIDOPROPYL PG-DIMONIUM CHLORIDE PHOSPHATE	977162530
FRAGRANCE	999999999
SODIUM LAURETH SULFATE	1335724
SODIUM LAURYL SULFATE	151213

Figure E-19 *An example of a Material Safety Data Sheet (MSDS) for shampoos (page 1).*

(Reprinted with permission of Clairol Inc.)

SODIUM LAURYL SULFATE	151213
COCAMIDOPROPYL BETAINE	61789400
SODIUM LAURETH SULFATE	1335724
SODIUM LAURYL SULFATE	151213
COCAMIDOPROPYL BETAINE	61789400
FRAGRANCE	999999999
SODIUM LAURETH SULFATE	1335724
DISODIUM LAUROAMPHODIACETATE	14350971
SODIUM TRIDECETH SULFATE	25446780
COCAMIDOPROPYL BETAINE	61789400
PEG-80 SORBITAN LAURATE	977090199
SODIUM LAURETH SULFATE	1335724
FRAGRANCE	999999999
COCAMIDOPROPYL BETAINE	61789400
SODIUM LAURETH SULFATE	1335724
SODIUM LAURYL SULFATE	151213
FRAGRANCE	999999999
SODIUM LAUROYL SARCOSINATE	137166
FRAGRANCE	999999999

Section III - Physical/Chemical Characteristics
Specific Gravity (H_2O = 1): 0.9-1.2

Solubility in Water: Highly miscible.

pH: 4 - 7

Appearance and Odor: Fragranced liquids or pourable emulsions.

Section IV - Fire and Explosion Hazard Data
Flashpoint: >200⁰   **Unit:** Fahrenheit   **Type:** Not applicable.

Method: closed cup

Fire Fighting Procedures:
Extinguish fires with ABC all-purpose extinguisher. The type of extinguisher used should be in conformance with local fire regulations. Fire fighters should use self contained breathing apparatus in enclosed areas.

Unusual Fire and Explosion Hazards:
None.

Physical Hazards
None.

Section V - Reactivity Data
Stability: Stable.

Conditions to Avoid: None.

Incompatibility (Materials ot Avoid): Not applicable.

Hazardous Decomposition or ByProducts: None.

Section VI- Health Hazards and Hazard Data
The TLV of the mixture has not been established.
1. Effects of Acute Accidental Exposure

Eye Contact: Eye irritant.

Skin Contact: Potential skin irritant.

Inhalation: Not applicable.

Ingestion: Slightly toxic.

Figure E-20 *An example of a Material Safety Data Sheet (MSDS) for shampoos (page 2).*
(Reprinted with permission of Clairol Inc.)

2. Effects of Chronic Exposure

National Toxicology Program studies on diethanolamine itself and fatty acid condensates containing free diethanolamine (DEA) (lauramide and cocamide diethanolamines) indicated an increased incidence of kidney and/or liver tumors in mice dermally exposed for their lifetime. The significance of these findings and their potential relevance to humans are not clear and further studies are in progress. Diethanolamine or its condensates did not induce tumor in rats. In the interim, the US CIR, which had previously considered these materials as "safe as used", has expressed reservation over NTP's conclusions and saw no need to revise its conclusion until several outstanding questions on the NTP methodology are answered. For purposes of chronic exposure under the OSHA Hazard Communication Standard, this is an untested mixture. These products have been used extensively by consumers and Worldwide Beauty Care is not aware of any significant adverse effects. Target Organs: These products contain ingredients which have been shown to affect tissues or organs when fed at high levels of exposure in animal studies not encountered in normal use. Target Organs Identified in animal studies are as follows: Alcohol Denat.: Liver, eye, CNS, reproductive. Glycerin: Kidney, liver. Propylene Glycol: CNS.

3. Carcinogen Status:

OSHA: No NTP: No IARC: No

4. Route of Entry:

Inhalation: No Ingestion: Yes Skin: Yes

5. Pre-existing dermatitis would likely be made worse by exposure to these products.

6. Emergency and First Aid Procedures

Eye Contact:	Remove contact lenses,if used. Flush immediately with plenty of water for 15 minutes. Get medical attention IMMEDIATELY.
Skin Contact:	If spilled,wash skin immediately with soap and water (do not use solvents). Change into clean clothing. If skin reaction develops,contact dermatologist.
Inhalation:	Remove person to fresh air. Increase ventilation.
Ingestion:	Rinse out mouth with water and administer large amounts of milk. Contact Poison Control Center.

Section VII - Precautions for Safe Handling and Use

Steps to be taken in Case Material is released or Spilled:

Contain spill and promptly clean up. Flush with water and wipe with towel or rinse to drain. Floor can be slippery when wet.

Waste Disposal Method:

Products covered by this MSDS are considered non-hazardous waste according to RCRA. Disposable should be in accordance with all applicable Local,State and Federal Regulations.

Precautions to be Taken in Handling and Storage:

Store products in even,normal temperatures. Keep containers tightly closed.

Section VIII - Control Measures

Ventilation:

Exhaust system ventilation should be adequate to avoid buildup of vapors.

Hand Protection:

Use impervious gloves to avoid possible skin reaction.

Eye Protection:

Avoid contact with eyes. Use protective eyewear,if splashing is possible.

Other Types of Protection:

Not applicable.

Respiratory Protection:

Avoid inhalation.

Work Hygienic Practices:

Always follow good hygienic work practices. Avoid eye,clothing,and prolonged skin contact with products. In case of contact,rinse thoroughly with water. Promptly clean up all spills.

Section IX - Transportation Information

DOT Class: Not regulated.	**IMDG:**Not regulated.	**IATA/ICAO:**Not regulated.

Figure E-21 *An example of a Material Safety Data Sheet (MSDS) for shampoos (page 3).*

(Reprinted with permission of Clairol Inc.)

Material Safety Data Sheet-PPD

MSDS:00008

Date Approved:
Worldwide Beauty Care
(Clairol, Inc.; Duart Labs; Redmond Products, Inc.)
Bristol-Myers Squibb Company
One Blachley Road
Stamford, CT 06922

Emergency Telephone Number:
(203) 357-5678

Transportation Emergency:
Call Chemtrec 1-800-424-9300

This sheet has been prepared in accordance with the Requirements of the OSHA Hazard Communication Standard, 29 CFR 1910.1200.

▼

Section I - Categorization

Product Category: Conditioners

Pertinent Text: Fragranced emulsions designed to enhance the appearance and feel of hair, increase hair body or suppleness, facilitate styling, improve gloss or sheen and improve the texture of hair.

Product Names: Aussie Conditioners, Color Hold Conditioner, Condition 3-In-1 Detangler & Beauty Pack, Daily Defense Conditioners, Frizz Control Taming Conditioner, Herbal Essences Conditioners, Jazzing Hair Color Shade 10, L'Image Conditioner, Loving Care Conditioner, Herbal Essences Hair Color After-Treatment, Miss Clairol Revitalizing Treatment, Motif Conditioner, Natural Instincts Treatment & Conditioner, Nice 'N Easy Conditioner, Revitalique Conditioner, Shimmer Lights Conditioner, Silk & Silver After Rinse Conditioner, Summer Blonde After Sun Conditioner, Textures & Tones 1 Minute Reconstructive Conditioner, Ultress & Ultimate Blonde Conditioner, Vitapointe Hair Treatment, Herbal Essence Conditioners , Renewal Conditioners, Aussie 3 Minute Miracle, Color ProTec Conditioner, Infusium 23 Pro-Vitamin Hair Treatment

▼

Section II - Ingredients Identity/Exposure Limits

Conditioners generally contain the following hazardous ingredients (1% concentration or greater; 0.1% for carcinogens):

CTFA Name	CAS Number
PROPYLENE GLYCOL	57556
ISOPROPYL ALCOHOL	67630
EXPOSURE LIMIT:400 ppm TLV, PEL, 500 ppm STEL	
ETHOXYDIGLYCOL	111900
GLYCERIN	56815
EXPOSURE LIMIT:AS A MIST 10 mg/m3 TLV, 15 mg/m3 TOTAL: 5 mg/m3 RESPIRABLE OSHA PEL	
STEARALKONIUM CHLORIDE	122190
HYDROLYZED COLLAGEN	92113310
PVP	9003398
CETEARYL ALCOHOL	67762270
ACETAMIDE MEA	142267
CETYL ALCOHOL	36653824
HYDROXYETHYLCELLULOSE	9004620
POLYSORBATE 20	9005645
HEXYLENE GLYCOL	107415
EXPOSURE LIMIT:25 ppm CEILING ACGIH	
SORBITOL	50704
CETYL ALCOHOL	36653824
MINERAL OIL	8012951
EXPOSURE LIMIT:5 mg/m3 TLV, PEL AS AN OIL MIST	
CETYL ESTERS	8002231
CITRIC ACID	77929

Figure E-22 *An example of a Material Safety Data Sheet* (MSDS) *for conditioners (page 1).*
(Reprinted with permission of Clairol Inc.)

POLYQUATERNIUM-10	53568664
STEARYL ALCOHOL	112925
DICETYLDIMONIUM CHLORIDE	1812539
PEG-150 DISTEARATE	9005087
EXPOSURE LIMIT:10 mg/m3 TLV	
PEG-100 STEARATE	90044993G
GLYCERYL STEARATE	31566311
EXPOSURE LIMIT:10 mg/m3 TLV	
HYDROLYZED COLLAGEN	92113310
PEG-40 STEARATE	9004993G
EXPOSURE LIMIT:10 mg/m3 TLV	
CETEARYL ALCOHOL	67762270
POLYQUATERNIUM-10	53568664
GLYCOL STEARATE	111604
POLYQUATERNIUM-6	26062793
HYDROLYZED COLLAGEN	92113310
AMODIMETHICONE	977091647
HYDROXYETHYLCELLULOSE	9004620
POLYQUATERNIUM-4	977086762
CETRIMONIUM CHLORIDE	112027
C12-15 ALKYL BENZOATE	68411278
TRIBEHENIN	18641571
QUATERNIUM-18	61789808
MYRISTYL MYRISTATE	3234853
CETEARYL ALCOHOL	67762270
BEHENTRIMONIUM METHOSULFATE	81646131
CETETH-2	5274613
DIMETHICONE	9006659
HYDROLYZED COLLAGEN	92113310
CETEARYL ALCOHOL	67762270
DISODIUM WHEATGERMAMPHODIACETATE	977169304
2,2,4-TRIMETHYL-1,3-PENTANEDIOL	144194
LINOLEAMIDOPROPYL DIMETHYLAMINE DIMER DILINOLEATE	125804106
PEG-20 ALMOND GLYCERIDES	124046500
CYCLOMETHICONE	69430246
QUATERNIUM-18	61789808
TRIMETHYLSILYLAMODIMETHICONE	977088826
CYCLOPENTASILOXANE	541026
CYCLOMETHICONE	69430246
DIMETHICONE	9006659
DICETYLDIMONIUM CHLORIDE	1812539
BEHENTRIMONIUM CHLORIDE	17301530
PHENYL TRIMETHICONE	2116849
QUATERNIUM-84	977172261
AMODIMETHICONE	977091647
PVP	9003398
KAOLIN	1332587
DIMETHICONE COPOLYOL MEADOWFOAMATE	157479511
PEG-12 DISTEARATE	977055074
SODIUM COCOAMPHOPROPIONATE	68988636
STEARETH-21	977080811
CETEARETH-20	68439496

Figure E–23 *An example of a Material Safety Data Sheet* (MSDS) *for conditioners* (page 2).
(Reprinted with permission of Clairol Inc.)

ᒬᒋ

Section III - Physical/Chemical Characteristics
Specific Gravity (H$_2$O = 1):0.8-1.15

Solubility in Water: Poor. Dispersible in water.

pH: N/A

Appearance and Odor: Mild fragranced liquids,cremes,pourable emulsions.

ᒬᒋ

Section IV - Fire and Explosion Hazard Data
Flashpoint: N/A   **Unit:** N/A   **Method:** Not applicable.   **Type:**Not applicable.

Fire Fighting Procedures:
Extinguish fires with ABC all-purpose extinguisher. The type of extinguisher used should be in conformance with local fire regulations. Fire fighters should use self contained breathing apparatus in enclosed areas.

Unusual Fire and Explosion Hazards:
None.

Physical Hazards
None.

ᒬᒋ

Section V - Reactivity Data
Stability: Stable.

Conditions to Avoid: None.

Incompatibility (Materials ot Avoid): Not applicable.

Hazardous Decomposition or ByProducts: None.

ᒬᒋ

Section VI- Health Hazards and Hazard Data
The TLV of the mixture has not been established.

1. Effects of Acute Accidental Exposure

Eye Contact: Potential eye irritant.
Skin Contact: Non-irritating.
Inhalation: Not applicable.
Ingestion: Practically non toxic.

2. Effects of Chronic Exposure
For purposes of chronic exposure under the OSHA Hazard Communication Standard, this is an untested mixture. These products have been used extensively by consumers and Worldwide Beauty Care is not aware of any significant adverse effects. Target Organs: These products contain ingredients which have been shown to affect tissues or organs when fed at high levels of exposure in animal studies not encountered in normal use. Target Organs identified in animal studies are as follows: Glycerin: Kidney, Liver; Propylene Glycol: CNS; Isopropyl Alcohol: CNS.

3. Carcinogen Status:
OSHA: No NTP: No IARC: No

4. Route of Entry:
Inhalation: No Ingestion: Yes Skin: Yes

5. Pre-existing dermatitis would likely be made worse by exposure to these products.

6. Emergency and First Aid Procedures
Eye Contact: Remove contact lenses,if used. Flush immediately with plenty of water for 15 minutes. Get medical attention IMMEDIATELY.

Skin Contact: If spilled,wash skin immediately with soap and water (do not use solvents). Change into clean clothing. If allergic reaction develops,contact dermatologist.

Inhalation: Remove person to fresh air. Increase ventilation.

Ingestion: Rinse out mouth with water and administer large amounts of milk. Contact Poison Control Center.

Figure E-24 *An example of a Material Safety Data Sheet* (MSDS) *for conditioners (page 3).*

(Reprinted with permission of Clairol Inc.)

Section VII - Precautions for Safe Handling and Use
Steps to be taken in Case Material is released or Spilled:
Contain spill and promptly cleanup. Flush with copious amounts of water until floor is not slippery.
Waste Disposal Method:
Products covered by this MSDS,in their original form,are considered non-hazardous waste according to RCRA.
Additionally,disposal should be in accordance with all applicable Local,State and Federal regulations.
Precautions to be Taken in Handling and Storage:
None.

Section VIII - Control Measures
Ventilation:
Exhaust system ventilation should be adequate to avoid buildup of vapors.
Hand Protection:
Use impervious gloves to avoid possible skin reaction.
Eye Protection:
Avoid contact with eyes. Use protective eyewear,if splashing is possible.
Other Types of Protection:
Not applicable.
Respiratory Protection:
Avoid inhalation.
Work Hygienic Practices:
Always follow good hygienic work practices. Avoid eye,clothing,and prolonged skin contact with products. In case
of contact,rinse thoroughly with water. Promptly clean up all spills.

Section IX - Transportation
Information

DOT Class: Not regulated.	**IMDG:**Not regulated.	**IATA/ICAO:**Not regulated.

Figure E–25 *An example of a Material Safety Data Sheet (MSDS) for conditioners (page 4).*

(Reprinted with permission of Clairol Inc.)

Material Safety Data Sheet-PPD

MSDS:00010

Date Approved:
Worldwide Beauty Care
(Clairol, Inc.; Duart Labs; Redmond Products, Inc.)
Bristol-Myers Squibb Company
One Blachley Road
Stamford, CT 06922

Emergency Telephone Number:
(203) 357-5678

Transportation Emergency:
Call Chemtrec 1-800-424-9300

This sheet has been prepared in accordance with the Requirements of the OSHA Hazard Communication Standard, 29 CFR 1910.1200.

▼

Section I - Categorization

Product Category: Flammable Aerosol Hair Sprays/Dry Shampoos
Pertinent Text: A concentrated liquid in an alcoholic/water base containing resins, conditioners and fragrance delivered in a propellant system.
Product Names: Condition 3-In-1 Hairsprays, Daily Defense Hairspray, PSSST, Sheer Mist Hairspray, Vitalis Hair Spray, Aussie Hairsprays, Color Protec Finishing Spray

▼

Section II - Ingredients Identity/Exposure Limits

Flammable Aerosol Hair Sprays/Dry Shampoos generally contain the following hazardous ingredients (1% concentration or greater; 0.1% for carcinogens):

CTFA Name	CAS Number
ALCOHOL DENAT.	64175
EXPOSURE LIMIT:1000 ppm TLV, PEL (ETHYL ALCOHOL)	
ETHYL ESTER OF PVM/MA COPOLYMER	67724930
DIMETHYL ETHER	115106
PROPANE	74986
EXPOSURE LIMIT:1000 PPM PEL, ACGIH ASPHYXIANT	
ISOBUTANE	75285
PROPANE	74986
EXPOSURE LIMIT:1000 PPM PEL, ACGIH ASPHYXIANT	
ISOBUTANE	75285
HYDROFLUOROCARBON 152A	75376
ISOBUTANE	75285
OCTYLACRYLAMIDE/ACRYLATES COPOLYMER	977131411
DIMETHYL ETHER	115106
VA/CROTONATES/VINYL NEODECANOATE COPOLYMER	55353214
ALCOHOL DENAT.	64175
EXPOSURE LIMIT:1000 ppm TLV, PEL (ETHYL ALCOHOL)	
PHENYL TRIMETHICONE	2116849
ALUMINUM STARCH OCTENYLSUCCINATE	9087610
HYDROFLUOROCARBON 152A	75376
DIGLYCOL/CHDM/ISOPHTHALATES/SIP COPOLYMER	999000483
OCTYLACRYLAMIDE/ACRYLATES/BUTYLAMINOETHYL METHACRYLATE COPOLYMER	708010879
ACRYLATES COPOLYMER	25085692

▼

Section III - Physical/Chemical Characteristics

Specific Gravity (H$_2$O = 1): Concentrate: 0.79-0.83
pH: N/A
Solubility in Water: Slightly soluble.
Appearance and Odor: Fragranced spray.

Figure E-26 *An example of a Material Safety Data Sheet* (MSDS) *for aerosol hair sprays (page 1).*
(Reprinted with permission of Clairol Inc.)

Section IV - Fire and Explosion Hazard Data

Flashpoint: Concentrate: 51-71 **Unit:** Fahrenheit

Type: For products containing alcohol.

Method: closed cup

Fire Fighting Procedures:
Extinguish fires with ABC all-purpose extinguisher. The type of extinguisher used should be in conformance with local fire regulations. Fire fighters should use self contained breathing apparatus in enclosed areas.

Unusual Fire and Explosion Hazards:
Product will flash or sustain a flame if exposed to fire, heat or ignition source at or below room temperature.

Physical Hazards
Flammable aerosol. Contents under pressure. Concentrate: Flammable liquid.

Section V - Reactivity Data

Stability: Stable.
Conditions to Avoid: Open flames; heat and ignition sources.
Incompatibility (Materials ot Avoid): None.
Hazardous Decomposition or ByProducts: May form toxic materials (carbon dioxide and carbon monoxide).

Section VI- Health Hazards and Hazard Data
The TLV of the mixture has not been established.
1. Effects of Acute Accidental Exposure

Eye Contact: Potential eye irritant.
Skin Contact: Irritation unlikely. Contact with propellant may cause frostbite.
Inhalation: Respiratory symptoms may occur due to inadequate ventilation. High concentration of propellants may induce anesthesia or anoxia.
Ingestion: Not likely to occur. Ingestion of 2 or more ounces of product containing high level of alcohol may result in depression and alcohol intoxication.

2. Effects of Chronic Exposure
For purposes of chronic exposure under the OSHA Hazard Communication Standard, these are untested mixtures. Aerosol hair spray formulations using a variety of resins and solvent-propellant systems have been tested for safety by Worldwide Beauty Care and industry-sponsored animal studies. There is no evidence in these studies that ingredients used in these products are harmful to general health or cause adverse effects on the respiratory system. Target Organs: Alcohol Denat.: Liver, CNS, Eye and Reproductive.

3. Carcinogen Status:
OSHA: No NTP: No IARC: No

4. Route of Entry:
Inhalation: Yes Ingestion: Yes Skin: Yes

5. Pre-existing dermatitis would likely be made worse by exposure to these products. Bronchitis may be aggravated by irritant vapors.

6. Emergency and First Aid Procedures

Eye Contact: Remove contact lenses, if used. Flush immediately with plenty of water for 15 minutes. Get medical attention IMMEDIATELY.
Skin Contact: If spilled, wash skin immediately with soap and water (do not use solvents). Change into clean clothing. If skin reaction develops, contact dermatologist.
Inhalation: Remove person to fresh air. Increase ventilation.
Ingestion: Rinse out mouth with water and administer large amounts of milk. Contact Poison Control Center.

Section VII - Precautions for Safe Handling and Use
Steps to be taken in Case Material is released or Spilled:
Avoid ignition sources. Material is flammable. Contain spill and promptly clean up. Flush with water. Floor can be

Figure E-27 *An example of a Material Safety Data Sheet (MSDS) for aerosol hair sprays (page 2).*

(Reprinted with permission of Clairol Inc.)

slippery when wet.
Waste Disposal Method:
These products are considered hazardous according to RCRA. Disposal should be in accordance with all applicable Local,State and Federal Regulations.
Precautions to be Taken in Handling and Storage:
Products under pressure. Do not puncture or incinerate. Do not store at temperature above 120 F or use near fire or flame. Keep out of reach of children.

Section VIII - Control Measures
Ventilation:
Exhaust system ventilation should be adequate to avoid buildup of vapors.
Hand Protection:
Use impervious gloves to avoid possible skin reaction.
Eye Protection:
Avoid contact with eyes. Use protective eyewear,if splashing is possible.
Other Types of Protection:
Not applicable.
Respiratory Protection:
Avoid inhalation.
Work Hygienic Practices:
Always follow good hygienic work practices. Avoid eye,clothing,and prolonged skin contact with products. In case of contact,rinse thoroughly with water. Promptly clean up all spills.

Section IX - Transportation
Information

DOT Class: Consumer Commodity ORM-D	**IMDG:**Aerosols 2.1 UN 1950 Limited Quantities	**IATA/ICAO:**Consumer Commodity Class: 9, ID 8000 Packing Instructions 910

Figure E–28 *An example of a Material Safety Data Sheet* (MSDS) *for aerosol hair sprays* (*page 3*).
(Reprinted with permission of Clairol Inc.)

Material Safety Data Sheet-PPD

MSDS:00011

Date Approved:
Worldwide Beauty Care
(Clairol, Inc.; Duart Labs; Redmond Products, Inc.)
Bristol-Myers Squibb Company
One Blachley Road
Stamford, CT 06922

Emergency Telephone Number: **Transportation Emergency:**
(203) 357-5678   Call Chemtrec 1-800-424-9300

This sheet has been prepared in accordance with the Requirements of the OSHA Hazard Communication Standard, 29 CFR 1910.1200.

▼

Section I - Categorization

Product Category: Non-Aerosol (Pump) Hair Sprays
Pertinent Text: Flammable alcoholic fragranced liquids.
Product Names: Clairmist, Color Protec Spritz, Condition 3-In-1 Hairsprays, Condition 3-In-1 Sculpting Spritz, Herbal Essences Hairspray, Herbal Essences Spritz, Infusium Hairspray, Daily Defense Hairspray, Aussie Mega Styling Spray, Vitalis Non-Aerosol Hairspray, Final Net Hairspray, Aussie Sprunch Spray

▼

Section II - Ingredients Identity/Exposure Limits
Non-Aerosol (Pump) Hair Sprays generally contain the following hazardous ingredients (1% concentration or greater; 0.1% for carcinogens):

CTFA Name	CAS Number
PROPYLENE GLYCOL	57556
ISOPROPYL ALCOHOL	67630
EXPOSURE LIMIT:400 PPM TLV, PEL 500 PPM STEL	
ALCOHOL DENAT.	64175
EXPOSURE LIMIT:1000 PPM TLV, PEL (ETHYL ALCOHOL)	
ETHYL ESTER OF PVM/MA COPOLYMER	67724930
AMINOMETHYL PROPANOL	124685
OCTYLACRYLAMIDE/ACRYLATES COPOLYMER	977131411
ACRYLATES/ACRYLAMIDE COPOLYMER	26062566
VA/CROTONATES/VINYL NEODECANOATE COPOLYMER	55353214
ALCOHOL DENAT.	64175
EXPOSURE LIMIT:1000 PPM TLV, PEL (ETHYL ALCOHOL)	
DIMETHICONE COPOLYOL	64365237
ALCOHOL DENAT.	64175
EXPOSURE LIMIT:1000 PPM TLV, PEL (ETHYL ALCOHOL)	
DIGLYCOL/CHDM/ISOPHTHALATES/SIP COPOLYMER	999000483
OCTYLACRYLAMIDE/ACRYLATES/BUTYLAMINOETHYL METHACRYLATE COPOLYMER	70801079
PVP/VA COPOLYMER	25086899
ALCOHOL DENAT.	64175
EXPOSURE LIMIT:1000 PPM TLV, PEL (ETHYL ALCOHOL)	
ACRYLATES COPOLYMER	25085692

▼

Section III - Physical/Chemical Characteristics

Specific Gravity (H$_2$O = 1):0.80-0.84   **pH:**   N/A

Solubility in Water: Slightly soluble.   **Appearance and Odor:**   Clear alcoholic liquid. Mildly fragranced.

Figure E-29 *An example of a Material Safety Data Sheet (MSDS) for non-aerosol pump hair sprays (page 1).*
(Reprinted with permission of Clairol Inc.)

M

Section IV - Fire and Explosion Hazard Data

Flashpoint:	52-65	**Unit:**	Fahrenheit	**Type:**	For products containing alcohol.
		Method:	closed cup		

Fire Fighting Procedures:
Extinguish fires with ABC all-purpose extinguisher. The type of extinguisher used should be in conformance with local fire regulations. Fire fighters should use self contained breathing apparatus in enclosed areas.

Unusual Fire and Explosion Hazards:
Product will flash or sustain a flame if exposed to fire,heat or ignition source at or below room temperature.

Physical Hazards
Flammable liquids.

Re

Section V - Reactivity Data

Stability: Stable.
Conditions to Avoid: Open flames; heat and ignition sources.
Incompatibility (Materials ot Avoid): None.
Hazardous Decomposition or ByProducts: May form toxic materials (carbon dioxide and carbon monoxide).

Ne

Section VI- Health Hazards and Hazard Data
The TLV of the mixture has not been established.

1. Effects of Acute Accidental Exposure

Eye Contact: Eye irritant.
Skin Contact: Non-irritating.
Inhalation: Respiratory symptoms may occur due to inadequate ventilation.
Ingestion: Moderately toxic. May cause strong burning sensation. Ingestion of 2 or more ounces of product containing high level of alcohol may result in depresion and alcohol intoxication.

2. Effects of Chronic Exposure
For purposes of chronic exposure under the OSHA Hazard Communication Standard, this is an untested mixture. These products have been used extensively by consumers and Worldwide Beauty Care is not aware of any significant adverse effects. Target Organs: These products contain an ingredient which has been shown to affect tissues or organs under high levels of exposure in animal studies not encountered in normal use. Alcohol: Liver, CNS, eye and reproductive.

3. Carcinogen Status:
OSHA: No NTP: No IARC: No

4. Route of Entry:
Inhalation: Yes Ingestion: Yes Skin: Yes

5. Pre-existing dermatitis would likely be made worse by exposure to these products. Bronchitis may be aggravated by irritant vapors.

6. Emergency and First Aid Procedures

Eye Contact: Remove contact lenses,if used. Flush immediately with plenty of water for 15 minutes. Get medical attention IMMEDIATELY.
Skin Contact: If spilled,wash skin immediately with soap and water (do not use solvents). Change into clean clothing. If skin reaction develops,contact dermatologist.
Inhalation: Remove person to fresh air. Increase ventilation.
Ingestion: Rinse out mouth with water and administer large amounts of milk. Contact Poison Control Center.

▼

Section VII - Precautions for Safe Handling and Use
Steps to be taken in Case Material is released or Spilled:
Avoid ignition sources. Material is flammable. Contain spill and promptly clean up. Flush with water. Floor can be slippery when wet.

Figure E-30 *An example of a Material Safety Data Sheet* (MSDS) *for non-aerosol pump hair sprays (page 2).*
(Reprinted with permission of Clairol Inc.)

Waste Disposal Method:
Products covered by this MSDS,in their original form,are considered non-hazardous waste according to RCRA (40 CFR 261.21(a)(1)). Additionally,disposal should be in accordance with all applicable Local,State and Federal regulations.

Precautions to be Taken in Handling and Storage:
FLAMMABLE! Keep away from fire and flames. Keep containers closed. Follow flammable liquid storage requirements. Keep away from radiators and heat. Store in a room with even,normal temperatures,away from heating elements.

Section VIII - Control Measures

Ventilation:
Exhaust system ventilation should be adequate to avoid buildup of vapors.

Hand Protection:
Use impervious gloves to avoid possible skin reaction.

Eye Protection:
Avoid contact with eyes. Use protective eyewear,if splashing is possible.

Other Types of Protection:
Not applicable.

Respiratory Protection:
Avoid inhalation.

Work Hygienic Practices:
Always follow good hygienic work practices. Avoid eye,clothing,and prolonged skin contact with products. In case of contact,rinse thoroughly with water. Promptly clean up all spills.

Section IX - Transportation Information

DOT Class:	IMDG:	IATA/ICAO:
Over 16 oz. containers: Ethyl Alcohol Solutions 3, UN1170, PG II, 16 oz. containers and under: Consumer Commodity ORM-D	Over 16 oz. containers: Ethyl Alcohol Solutions 3.2 UN1170, PGII, Under 16 oz containers: Ethyl Alcohol Solutions, 3.2 UN1170, PGII, Limited Quantities	Over 16 oz. containers: Ethyl Alcohol Solutions, 3, UN1170, PGII, Packing Instructions 305, Under 16 oz. containers: Consumer Commodity, Class 9, ID8000, Packing Instructions 910

Figure E–31 *An example of a Material Safety Data Sheet (MSDS) for non-aerosol pump hair sprays (page 3).*
(Reprinted with permission of Clairol Inc.)

Kenra, LLC 6501 Julian Ave., Indianapolis, IN 46219

Product Name　　VOLUME SPRAY (80% VOC)

Product Description　Finishing Aid

KENRA
CLASSIC. QUALITY. HAIRCARE.

| **MSDS Number:** | 16100 | **Revision Date:** | 01-Nov-00 |

Section 2 - Hazardous Ingredients / Identity Information

Hazardous Components	CAS Number	TLV or PEL	Other Limits	Percentage
Ethanol	64-17-5	N/A	N/A	N/A
Aminomethyl Propanol	124-68-5	N/A	N/A	N/A
Isobutane	68476-85-7	N/A	N/A	N/A
Ethane,1,1-Difluoro-	75-37-6	N/A	N/A	N/A

Section 3 - Physical/Chemical Characteristics

Boiling Point　@760mmHg 173-F　　**Specific Gravity H20 = 1**　@70-F = .806-820

Vapor Pressure (mm Hg.)　N/A　　**Melting Point**　N/A

Vapor Density (AIR = 1)　>1　　**Evaporation Point(Butyl Acetate = 1)**　N/A

Solubility in Water　Soluble

Appearance and Odor　Clear light straw liquid / characteristic odor

Section 4 - Fire and Expolsion Hazard

Flash Point (Method Used)	Flammable Limits	LEL	UEL
-30 - F	N/A	N/A	N/A

Extinguishing Media

Carbon Dioxide, Foam, Dry Chemical, Water

Special Fire Fighting Procedures

Keep temperature of containers below 120-F by spraying with water until the fire has been extinguish

Unusual Fire and Explosion Hazards

Containers may rupture and release flammable liquids and/or gases if exposed to heat or fire.

Section 5 - Reactvity Data

Stability	Unstable ☐	**Conditions to Avoid**
	Stable ☑	Do not store containers in direct sunlight or where conditions will heat them above 120-F.

Incompatibilty (Materials to Avoid)

Do not mix with strong oxidizers.

Hazardous Decomposition or Byproducts

Normal products of combustion.

Hazardous Polymerization	May Occur ☐	**Conditions to Avoid**
	May Not Occur ☑	N/A

Figure E-32 An example of a Material Safety Data Sheet (MSDS) for non-aerosol pump hair sprays (page 1).
(Reprinted with permission of Kenra LLC.)

Section 6 - Health Hazard Data

Routes of Entry	Inhalation ?	Skin ?	Ingestion ?
	☐	☐	☑

Health Hazards (Acute and Chronic)

Prolonged skin contact may cause dermatitis in sensitive individuals.

Carcinogenicity	NTP	IARC	OSHA
	☐	☐	☐

Signs and Symptoms of Exposure

Redness, stinging, or burning of the skin.

Medical Conditions Generally Aggravated by Exposure

N/A

Emergency and First Aid Procedures

Wash from skin or eyes with large amounts of water. If irritation occurs, consult a physician.

Section 7 - Precautions for Safe Handling and Use

Steps to be Taken in Case Material is Released or Spilled

Leaking cans should be placed in open containers, outdoors, away from any source of ignition, until all pressure has been released.

Waste Disposal Method

Bury or incinerate in approved disposal Facilites and accordance with Ferderal, State and Local reg.

Precautions to be Taken in Handling and Storage

N/A

Other Precautions

N/A

Section 8 - Control Measures

Respiratory Protection (Specify Type)

NIOSH/MSHS - approved organic vapor respirator when vapors are generated above the permissable limit.

Ventilation (Specify Type: Local Exhaust, Mechanical, Special, Other)

Local exhaust to control to recommended P.E.L.

Gloves (Specify Type)	Eye
PVC,Rubber,Plastic, Neoprene	Chemical goggles

Other Protective Clothing or Equipment

Coveralls, aprons, boots, as necessary to prevent skin contact.

Hygiene

Wash hands after use.

KENRA, LLC makes no warranty, express or implied, as to the accuracy, completeness or reliability of information contained here, except that such information is, to the best of our knowledge and belief, accurate as of the date indicated. We assume no responsibility for the application of this information or the consequences of its use.

Figure E-32 *An example of a Material Safety Data Sheet (MSDS) for non-aerosol pump hair sprays (page 2).*
(Reprinted with permission of Kenra LLC.)

Appendix F

Product Ingredients

COVERT CONTROL HOLDING SPRAY

Ingredients

SD Alcohol 40 - used to keep the resin blend in a liquid state until it is in place. The alcohol quickly evaporates and does not alter the pH of the hair in the process. When used in this manner it is not drying to the hair (a popular misconception).

Isobutane - the principal propellant . . . the thing that makes an aerosol an aerosol. It moves the contents from inside the container onto the hair. This is one of the new safe propellants. It is an element of natural gas.

Hydrofluorocarbon 152a - another non-VOC propellant. It gives hair spray the drying time stylists are accustomed to and it's better for our air. It costs more than the old propellants and more than the water/Dimethyl Ether systems that you see in the supermarket, but the performance is much superior.

Octylacrylamide/Acrylates/Butylaminoethyl Methacrylate Copolymer - can you imagine what chemists name their children? - this is nothing more than our resin blend . . . to hold the hair in place.

Aminomethyl Propanol - the emulsifying agent. This ingredient helps keep all the other ingredients mixed together.

Dimethicone Copolyol - keeps the resins flexible and soft on the hair shaft.

Phenyl Trimethicone - this is a very light oil used to keep our resin blend flexible once it is on the hair.

Triethyl Citrate - better known as citric acid. It works in our formula as a solvent and assists in keeping the resins soft.

Lauramide DEA - from vegetable oils, this common constituent of shampoo is also used to keep the resins soft and to hold the formulation in solution.

AMP Isostearoyl Hydrolyzed Wheat Protein - works both as a conditioner and to add extra body to the hair in a very natural way.

Fragrance - TRI's special "fugitive" fragrance. A sophisticated citric note with the ability to quickly disappear after application.

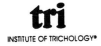

INSTITUTE OF TRICHOLOGY®

Figure F-1 A *list of ingredients for an aerosol hairspray.*
(Reprinted with permission of Tri, Institute of Trichology.)

TRI LIGHTS

Ingredients

Cyclomethicone - a silicone fluid oil from silica which is found abundantly in nature. It is a wonderful lubricant that effectively holds moisture within the hair. Cyclomethicone along with Dimethicone below, are the elements responsible for the shine. While they look like oils they don't feel greasy.

Isopropyl Palmitate - part of the shine package, this oil clings to the hair helping to hold the shine there. It comes from natural fats found in plants.

Dimethicone - the shine. Another good feature of Dimethicone and Cyclomethicone is low toxicity; they are almost never found to cause irritations or allergic reactions (unlike so many other ingredients in nature).

Octyl Methoxycinnamate - aren't you glad your mother didn't decide this would be a cute name. Actually, it is an acid found in cinnamon leaves that provides sunscreen protection for the hair. Researchers are questioning the value of sunscreens on hair, but until the final results are in, they can't hurt.

Propyl Paraben - an oil phase preservative commonly used because of its effectiveness against a very wide range of bacteria.

Technical Specifications

pH..none since there is no water in the product..

Available Sizes:

Net Weight ....1 oz.   (30 ML.)

- Biodegradable.
- Ingredients are derived from natural sources wherever possible.
- No animal ingredients were used in Tri Lights.
- No animal testing was used in the development of the product.

tri
INSTITUTE OF TRICHOLOGY•

Figure F-2 A *list of ingredients for a silicone conditioner.*
(Reprinted with permission of Tri, Institute of Trichology.)

GEL SPRAY

Ingredients

Water – purified and deionized, this is great water although you wouldn't like the taste without some mineral content. The CTFA recommends that ethical manufacturers only list it as "water", and that's precisely what we do.

Polyquaternium-10 – an antibacterial and conditioning agent. It does add some body while protecting the condition of the hair. It fights the growth of any bacteria that finds its way into the product.

PVP – The hold in Gel Spray. A resin similar to egg white. The film it forms adheres to the hair shaft.

Polysorbate-20 – an emulsifier commonly used in baby lotions. Used to stabilize oils in water - to make them mix.

Aloe Vera Extract – the untreated, "free run" juice of the aloe leaf. Its amino acids are part of the body building and conditioning package in this product.

Lemongrass Extract – an oil distilled from the leaves. (It tastes wonderful in Vietnamese food.) It is usually found in perfumes in the personal care industry, it acts as a carrier to fragrances.

Whole Wheat Protein – the premier conditioning factor in Gel Spray. It improves the body and shine of the hair.

Calendula Extract – from the floret of what is also called the marigold is derived this natural oil. The oil contains some natural resins which add to our body building package.

Balm Mint Extract – comes from a small evergreen tree. It is a very old cosmetic ingredient used to enhance body in the hair.

Carbomer-980 – an emulsifying and thickening agent. This is the gel in Gel Spray.

Triethanolamine – a moisture absorber used in making emulsions.

Methylparaben – a water phase preservative to prevent the growth of bacteria. It's approved for use in food.

Quaternium-15 – another part of the preservative package. It's antiseptic and germicide qualities make it widely used in the personal care industry.

Fragrance – smells very similar to another product in the TRI line, guess which one.

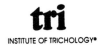

tri

INSTITUTE OF TRICHOLOGY®

Figure F-3 *A list of ingredients for a spray hair gel.*

(Reprinted with permission of Tri, Institute of Trichology.)

EXPRESS CONDITIONING DETANGLER

Ingredients

Water - the water in this product is wonderfully pure and clean. From a laboratory standpoint it is perfect. Lots of our competitors would attempt to disguise its first place position by floating herbs in it, calling it an herbal extract. We follow the suggestions of the CTFA, so on our label we call it – water.

Hydrolyzed Soy Protein - a vegetable protein from the versatile little soybean. Soy protein makes the hair more manageable. It has another plus – it's a moisturizer.

Polyquaternium-11 - an antibacterial and conditioning agent. It does add some body while protecting the condition of the hair.

Amodimethicone - a silicone fluid oil which is found abundantly in nature. It is a wonderful lubricant that effectively holds moisture within the hair. While amodimethicone looks like an oil it doesn't feel like one; it's not greasy.

Panthenol - an old friend in the hair care business. There are entire product lines based on this one ingredient. It is a member of the B-vitamin complex. Panthenol helps give the appearance of added body by swelling the hair shaft.

Hydrolyzed Keratin Protein - the stuff hair is made of. It naturally contains cystine, which as you know from Whole Wheat Shampoo Treatment, covalently bonds to the hair giving very long lasting conditioning effects.

Cocodimonium Hydroxypropyl Hydrolyzed Soy Protein - you thought we made a mistake and listed this ingredient twice. This is another form of soy protein. It is quite substantative in human hair and improves its condition. It links to damaged hair sites with an ionic bond.

Octyl Menthoxycinnamate - since Express Conditioning Detangler stays in the hair, we added a sunscreen. This one is found in cinnamon bark and hyacinth flower.

Biotin - another member of the B vitamin complex. In hair care products it is used to improve the texture of the product, it makes it creamier.

Chamomile Extract - from genuine German Chamomile. This herbal extract contains a volatile oil that has anti-inflammatory properties. Folk remedies have long called for its use in scalp problems.

Jojoba Oil - TRI was the first major manufacturer to use Jojoba oil in a hair care product many years ago, now Jojoba oil is a familiar hair care ingredient. We added it in this formula because of its extremely low melting point. It doesn't feel oily on the hair, but it helps to detangle and condition the hair.

tri
INSTITUTE OF TRICHOLOGY®

Figure F-4 *A list of ingredients for a leave-in conditioner.*
(Reprinted with permission of Tri, Institute of Trichology.)

WHOLE WHEAT CONDITIONING RINSE

Ingredients

Water - purified and deionized, this is great water, but it is just that - water. The CTFA suggests that ethical manufacturers only list it as "water" on all labels. That is exactly what we do.

Glyceryl Stearate - used in this formulation, it functions as a humectant, and emollient. This is the first of several conditioning elements you will see in this product. An interesting side note about Glyceryl Stearate is that it is frequently used on pasta and cereals to alter the texture and appearance. So, it is recognized as safe for consumption by the FDA.

Cetyl Alcohol - this one always confuses beginning label readers. When we think of alcohol we think of it as a liquid and we either drink it or use it to clean things with. At the time that cetyl alcohol goes into this product, it is a cream-colored, odorless flake. It is used as an emollient or another conditioning element. It gives a velvety feel to the skin and hair.

Hydrolyzed Wheat Protein - the premier conditioning factor in this rinse. It has been shown to covalently bond to the hair, providing some permanent conditioning effects. It improves the body and shine of the hair. We think it gives terrific manageability.

Panthenol - this is part of the water-soluble vitamin B complex. Panthenol is incorporated into this formulation to help give the hair the appearance of added body. Panthenol swells the hair shaft almost 10 times more than water does, and the effects last through several combings.

Birch Bark Extract - as an herbal medicine, it was used for years to heal sores externally. Today, it has found a place as a natural shine enhancer.

Cetrimonium Chloride - a conditioner used because of its antistatic properties.

Olive Oil - considered by chemists to be "the standard" for emollience. Olive oil is super stable and is a wonderful lubricant for hair care products.

Phenoxyethanol - a bacteria killer.

Methyl Paraben - a preservative used in foods, beverages, and hair care products. Methyl paraben is an important antioxidant.

Fragrance - a light, slightly citrus note that vanishes in the hair.

INSTITUTE OF TRICHOLOGY®

Figure F-5 *A list of ingredients for a conditioner.*
(Reprinted with permission of Tri, Institute of Trichology.)

WHOLE WHEAT SHAMPOO TREATMENT

Ingredients

Water - the water in this shampoo is purified and deionized, but we follow the labeling suggestions of the CTFA, so on our label it is just called - water.

Cocamide DEA - the main cleansing agent in our surfactant blend. It is derived from coconut oil. It is known for its gentle cleansing properties.

Cocamidopropyl Betaine - another portion of the surfactant blend. It also comes from coconut fatty acids. It has good conditioning and softening abilities.

Sodium Laureth Sulfate - this is a very mild, yet effective cleansing ingredient. In this particular blend of cleansing agents, it provides the rich sudsing.

Sodium C14-16 Olefin Sulfonate - yet another portion of our surfactant blend. This one is widely used in the industry; it's thought of as the "workhorse" of cleansing agents. A good, effective cleanser.

PVP - a body building agent. Gives hair the look and feel of increased volume.

Hydrolyzed Whole Wheat Protein - the prime conditioning element in this shampoo. Research suggests that the conditioning effects from this ingredient can be permanent.

Echinacea Extract - from the Purple Cone Flower comes this interesting herbal extract. It was used by American Indians to treat wounds and later by pharmacologists to treat eczema.

Chamomile Extract - from genuine German Chamomile. This herbal extract contains a volatile oil that has anti-inflammatory properties. Folk remedies have long called for its use in scalp and various skin conditions.

Wheat Germamidopropyl Betaine - from the heart of the wheat kernel - the "germ", comes this last portion of our surfactant blend. This particular one helps to modify the viscosity of the total product while naturally stabilizing foam.

Fragrance - following the TRI fragrance philosophy of light, fugitive fragrances, this one is present in such small quantities that it is hard to put your finger on. It has a bright, clean bouquet with a slightly sweet finish.

Grapefruit Seed Extract - a natural antiseptic and antibacterial agent from those little seeds you have always been careful not to eat.

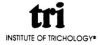

INSTITUTE OF TRICHOLOGY®

Figure F-6 A *list of ingredients for a shampoo.*
(Reprinted with permission of Tri, Institute of Trichology.)

Glossary/Index